Baby

Massage

A Comprehensive Guide for Parents and Instructors

HELEN McGUINNESS

 Hodder & Stoughton

A MEMBER OF THE HODDER HEADLINE GROUP

Orders: please contact Bookpoint Ltd, 130 Milton Park, Abingdon, Oxon OX14 4SB.
Telephone: (44) 01235 827720. Fax: (44) 01235 400454.
Lines are open from 9.00–6.00, Monday to Saturday, with a 24 hour message answering service.
You can also order through our website www.hodderheadline.co.uk

British Library Cataloguing in Publication Data
A catalogue record for this title is available from the British Library

ISBN 0 340 869283

First Published 2003

Impression number   10 9 8 7 6 5 4 3 2 1
Year   2007   2006   2005   2004   2003

Photographs by John Birdsall

Cover photo from Bubbles Photolibrary

Typeset by Phoenix Photosetting, Chatham, Kent
Printed in Great Britain for Hodder & Stoughton Educational, a division of Hodder Headline Plc, 338 Euston Road, London NW1 3BH by Trento

Foreword

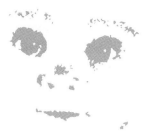

The Federation of Holistic Therapists was one of the first professional associations for therapists to recognise the value of the baby massage technique in the early 1990s. The last decade has seen an enormous growth in the demand for training in this field from therapists, midwives and health visitors as well as from parents themselves. At heart, the truth that baby massage illustrates, and which it has taken the medical profession so long to acknowledge, is that touch is incredibly important to human well-being. We are actually very tactile creatures and touch is the simplest form of communication for a baby to understand. This need does not diminish with age and we continue to feel the power of touch throughout our lives.

But, baby massage is not just for the benefit of the baby itself. As a mother I know that there are many myths surrounding the mother and baby relationship. Learning how to relate to this new unique person is not always easy or instinctive. Baby massage is a useful tool to help in the bonding process and I have heard of countless stories where baby massage has helped to achieve a better relationship and a more contented baby.

One of the benefits of this new book is its breadth, covering everything from baby development and communication through to advice on working with special needs infants and the integration of baby massage with other complementary therapy techniques. Though its appeal will be widespread, it will be ideal for the trainee practitioner no matter what their background.

Jacqueline Palmer
Chief Executive, Federation of Holistic Therapists (FHT)
Editor, *International Therapist* magazine

Massage has been a valued part of childcare in many cultures for hundreds of years. Baby massage has a positive impact on parents and the relationship with their baby. The simple routines allow them to express their love for their child through touch as well as relieving stress and helping to resolve minor ailments.

Baby Massage contains extensive chapters on anatomy and physiology and growth and development as well as the practical aspects of massage techniques.

Helen McGuinness has produced a comprehensive, user-friendly guide to baby massage for therapists, health care professionals and parents who wish to widen their knowledge base.

Jacqui Billingham
Midwife, Great Yarmouth Primary Health Care Trust

Acknowledgements

I would like to acknowledge and thank the following for helping to make this book possible.

To my husband Mark for his considerable help, love and support of my work, and especially for his constructive and valued contributions.

To Grace, our beautiful daughter who has taught me so much about baby massage.

To my parents Roy and Val for their understanding and support; and to my mother-in-law Daphne whose care of Grace was much needed at times in order to help me complete the book.

To GP Nathan Moss for his help, valued contributions and constructive feedback on the baby anatomy and physiology chapter.

To Vanessa Parker and Jasmin, Debbie Morgan-Clayton and Connor for so kindly providing their support and generous devotion of their time in helping to create the photographs for this book.

Preface

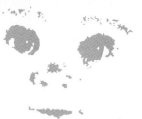

Baby massage, although part of daily life in some Eastern cultures, has only recently become a subject of great interest to parents, carers, health care professionals and holistic therapists alike.

VTCT, a leading Awarding Body of new Qualification Provision, designed a Qualification in Baby Massage Instruction in 1995. This Award was piloted and implemented at the Holistic Training Centre in 1996.

Since 1996, The Holistic Training Centre has trained a large number of baby massage instructors who now offer baby massage classes with groups and individuals in the community.

Word continues to spread of the benefits of baby massage throughout GP surgeries, midwives, health visitors and the health service.

I have had the great fortune to have been teaching baby massage to many parents out in the community since 1995, as well as members of my own family (including our daughter Grace who is a great fan of massage!). All of these people have all taught me a great deal about massage and its benefits.

This book proposes to address the need in the market for a more comprehensive and professional approach to this fascinating subject and I hope it will be valuable for parents, carers and instructors alike.

Helen McGuinness

Contents

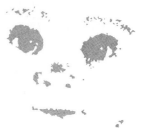

Introduction to Baby Massage 01

Baby massage is not a new idea, moreover it is one that is being re-discovered.

Baby massage is an art of nurturing which encourages loving communication between parents and their children, by encouraging positive physical contact, bonding and stimulation of a child's development.

The first few months after having a baby can be a challenging time for parents; massage can therefore play a vital role in enriching the lives of both the baby and its parents by bringing a sense of fulfilment, contentment and well-being.

Massaging babies has been part of traditional family life in eastern countries for centuries. However, despite the fact of the therapeutic benefits of massage on adults having long been established in the West, it is only within the last few decades that the benefits of massaging babies have become more recognised.

Massage has become one of the most popular treatment choices for adults seeking relief from stress and tension. Now, a growing number of parents are discovering that massaging their babies is an enjoyable way to nurture and bond with their babies, whilst improving the infant's responsiveness and overall health. Touch is as important to a baby's development as food.

The idea of baby massage was first introduced as a parenting tool in the mid- to late-1970s in the United States of America (USA) at a time when touch therapy and the intimacy of massaging children was unheard of.

It is through the work of pioneers such as Vimala McClure in the USA and Peter Walker in the United Kingdom (UK) that infant massage has progressed to help thousands of parents 'get in touch' with their babies.

Since the mid- to late-1990s baby massage has developed in popularity in the UK with greater emphasis on the importance of physical bonding and attachment between parent and baby. There is a growing awareness of the benefits of baby massage, as the focus shifts back to customary 'hands-on' practices of our ancestors that were previously abandoned in favour of progress.

Baby massage is a source of physical and emotional nourishment for both babies and their parents and is a form of mutual exchange. It is not another therapy; it is an opportunity for parents to share their love with their babies.

Cultural Differences in Baby Massage

Baby massage has been part of some cultures for thousands of years; for centuries families in the Far East have been using massage from birth as an important means of maintaining good health.

In eastern cultures it is something practised through the family, for the mother following the birth, and for the baby. Massage is part of a daily childcare routine in the East; babies are massaged daily by their grandmothers and then their mothers. Massage is thought to help protect the baby's skin, as well as encouraging them to relax and become more flexible.

The cultural differences in the East are quite different to the western approach, in that in the East massage is considered to be one of the principal means of strengthening the body, aiding healthy development and preventing disease.

The eastern culture recognises the importance of close skin and body contact as a natural daily custom. Many mothers in tribal, urban and rural eastern countries such as India, Africa, Asia, Nigeria and Uganda carry out their daily duties with their babies supported in slings. This has the advantage of babies being close to their mother's bodies and being able to experience the rhythm and movement of daily movements to stimulate their emotional and motor development.

Modern westernised practices are only recently rediscovering these 'positive touch' practices and learning the benefits of incorporating them into a western lifestyle. It is an unfortunate fact that a western lifestyle restricts parents from carrying their babies close to them at all times.

Babies rely on physical touch for their healthy development; the physical contact provided through a massage session provides both parent and baby with an opportunity for close physical contact to support the baby's emotional, physical and mental growth.

Modern Developments of Baby Massage

Baby massage instruction classes are now starting to become a regular feature in GP surgeries, hospitals, health clinics and the community, as midwives, health visitors, nursery nurses and massage therapists are embracing the skill.

Baby massage classes are starting to become an integral part of the help offered to parents in 'Healthy Start' Clinics' and Parentcraft classes run by midwives and health visitors under the National Health Service (NHS).

The 'Sure Start' scheme is a special government initiative which aims to promote the physical, intellectual and social development of children from birth to pre-school age. This scheme has already sponsored several Health Services (including ones in Liverpool and Great Yarmouth) in the promotion of baby massage classes throughout the community midwives, health visitors and nursery nurses.

Baby massage instruction, if not available through the NHS, is also being offered privately through a qualified instructor who may offer one-to-one tuition and group tuition, depending on the needs of the parents.

To contact a qualified baby massage instructor in your area please refer to the resource section at the back of this book.

The Role of a Baby Massage Instructor

Learning baby massage instruction is a special way of extending a massage therapist/health professional's skills, and can be a very rewarding experience in encouraging parents to massage their babies.

The role of a baby massage instructor is to educate and empower parents and carers on how to massage their babies. It provides a gentle intervention that supports and encourages them as they develop confidence in their skills.

It is important that the parents, and not the instructor, are encouraged to massage their babies in order that they can practice the skills at home for continuing benefit to the whole family. The beauty of baby massage lies in the fact that it is an innate skill present in all parents/carers. It is the baby massage instructor's role to nurture this skill.

It is a simple skill for parents to learn from a qualified instructor and one that does not require special talents or resources to continue. It is easy enough to be able to incorporate into the busiest of family lives, and is also a skill that may be developed and enjoyed by families throughout the generations.

Research on Baby Massage

There are many internet sites, which are easily accessible, relating to research information on baby massage; however these predominantly cover the effects of baby massage in relation to the care of pre-term or fragile infants. More research articles are available through USA websites as opposed to the UK, with one such site being www.infantmassage.com, which has a fairly extensive list of sources on research information.

Another source of research information, which again focuses on the effects of massage and touch with pre-term or fragile infants, is through the Neonatal Intensive Care Units (NICU). Their studies have resulted in findings, which show positive benefits for both babies and parents such as greater weight gain and shorter hospitalisation for the infant receiving massage. It also looks at the emergence of Kangaroo, or skin-to-skin practice, which in the main has been proven to have beneficial physiological and attachment outcomes. Further information can be accessed through NICU, the NHS in the UK or other main medical organisations worldwide. The internet again is usually the quickest method to access the information, although it can also be accessed manually through libraries.

One area of research related to the effects of baby massage concerns the subject of help with post-natal depression. Dr Vivette Glover, an expert in child stress and based at the Queen Charlotte's Hospital in London, spoke about the positive benefits resulting from a small study, which compared the results of mothers suffering from post-natal depression, some of whom massaged their babies, some of whom did not. She also called for more mothers to be educated in baby massage due to the positive outcomes. Further information on this research can be accessed through the Cochrane library (see below).

Internet sites which provide a wide range of research information on baby massage include Medline, more specifically Pubmed at www.ncbi.nih.gov/entrez/query.fcgi, which provides listings of research, medical, clinical and general. However; this is a subscription service and involves costs for both purchasing the information and also for compliance with copyright legislation.

The Cochrane library is an extensive and helpful source for information on baby massage research and related topics. It is a subscription service, although internet access is provided free in the UK through the NHS and can be accessed at www.nelh.nhs.uk/cochrane.asp.

Activity

Source and assimilate the various articles, discussions and research studies relating to baby massage from the above sources along with any additional sources you can find. Cross reference these items and comment on your findings. What is the general consensus and conclusions relating to the effects and results provided from the application of baby massage?

Questions for Review

1. When and why was baby massage introduced to the UK as a parenting tool?

_____

_____

_____

_____

_____

_____

_____

_____

_____

_____

_____

2. What are the main cultural differences towards baby massage between the East and West?

_____

_____

_____

_____

_____

_____

_____

_____

_____

_____

3. Explain the role of a baby massage instructor

_____

_____

_____

_____

_____

_____

The Benefits of 02
Baby Massage

Massage is a powerful sensory intervention that provides a wide range of physiological and psychosocial benefits for babies from birth through to childhood and beyond.

Massage for a baby begins in the uterus. The uterine contractions in labour stimulate the autonomic nervous system to signal a baby's respiratory system, and other internal systems prepare to function independently of its mother. Following birth, there is a period of great change in which a new relationship is formed and the demands of a new-born baby become a reality. Bonding with a new-born is not always a natural consequence and massage can help a parent to develop a deeper understanding of the importance of touch.

Baby massage can have profound benefits to the baby and its parents, and by taking the time to massage their child, a parent is helping to teach important qualities such as love, respect and caring.

The benefits of baby massage are reciprocal, in that whatever helps the baby also helps the parent, and whatever helps the parent aids the healthy development of the child.

By the end of this chapter you will be able to relate the following knowledge to your role as instructor/parent/carer:

* The physiological benefits of massage for babies
* The psychological value of massage to babies
* The benefits of baby massage for parents/carers
* The role and value of baby massage as a form of communication.

Benefits for Babies

Massage can help babies' bodies to release tension and stress that often arises from having to adapt to the world outside of the womb where they are nurtured and cradled.

Massage has many physiological benefits for babies:

* Stimulates a baby's circulation (increased blood flow ensures oxygen and nutrients reach baby's cells and tissues)
* Stimulates and strengthens a baby's immune system, through increased stimulation of the lymphatic circulation
* Aids digestion and elimination by activating relaxation responses (can help relieve colic and constipation)
* Encourages muscular co-ordination and joint flexibility
* Encourages faster weight gain (underweight babies can benefit by an increase in appetite)
* Promotes fuller and deeper respiration, increasing cell regeneration for growth and development
* Improves the appearance and texture of the skin (massaging a baby's skin with oil helps to nourish the skin and enhance absorption and elimination)
* Stimulation of the skin through massage increases the production of endorphins which helps to reduce pain and tension, and improves emotional well-being by elevating mood
* Improves sensory awareness due to tactile stimulation
* Stimulates the nervous system through stimulation of skin (speeds up myelination of nerves to enhance neurological and motor development)
* Babies delivered by Caesarean section benefit from massage as they don't get the cutaneous stimulation of the birth canal.

Psychological benefits of massage to babies include the following:

* Soothes and comforts, helping to relieve anxiety and trauma (effective in reducing the consequences of birth trauma)

✳ Stimulation of the skin through massage increases the production of endorphins, which helps to reduce pain and tension, and improves emotional well-being by elevating mood

✳ Reduces tension, restlessness and irritability

✳ Promotes relaxation and helps induce sleep (deeper and longer)

✳ Helps teach babies to experience relaxation and to self-calm

✳ Massage helps to teach babies about their body

✳ Gives babies reassurance through skin contact

✳ Improves sensory awareness due to tactile stimulation

✳ Promotes emotional security and a healthy body image through the development of body awareness

✳ Helps foster parent–baby bonding due to intimate interaction time

✳ Teaches babies about communication (helps build social skills)

✳ Increases vocalisation; assisting in speech and language development

✳ Powerful demonstration of unconditional love.

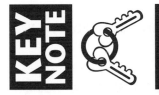

KEY NOTE   Babies, whether premature, underweight or full term can benefit from massage, in fact medical research has shown that massaging premature babies produces better weight gain and increased growth and development.

Benefits for Parents

Massage provides the focus for a warm and loving relationship with their child and is a means of parents expressing their love and developing a better understanding of their child.

Massage has many benefits for parents in that it:

✳ Deepens and strengthens the relationship between a baby and its parents by encouraging bonding and attachment (reciprocal process)

✳ The father or other primary carer, such as a grandparent, can enjoy the same emotional fulfilment as the mother, and can increase bonding. A baby learns that the father can also offer physical and emotional support

❉ Massaging a baby benefits the breast-feeding mother by enhancing the secretion of prolactin, which is essential for milk production

❉ Helps parents relax

❉ Helps parents to read baby cues/non-verbal signs

❉ Helps parents to learn about their baby and to interpret their needs and desires

❉ Enhances communication and builds mutual respect

❉ Helps increase confidence and self-esteem in parenting role

❉ Develops confidence of parents in handling their baby

❉ Fosters feelings of comfort, trust, enjoyment and security

❉ Can help reduce stress in a baby and its parents, helping them both to cope more easily

❉ Increases parents' ability to help relax baby in times of stress/distress

❉ Provides a period of mutual pleasure and focused time and attention for both baby and parents to enjoy

❉ Helps parents to become more aware and understanding of the baby's needs, as the massage becomes a form of loving communication

❉ Provides a special time for intimacy

❉ Provides a positive parenting tool for parents that helps nurture their baby's physical and emotional development.

The importance of Baby Massage as a form of communication

Massage is an effective form of loving communication and through massaging, parents can learn a great deal about their babies. A great deal of communication takes place through eye contact and this should be reinforced throughout the massage as much as possible.

Communicating with a baby involves touching, holding, rocking, talking, active listening and learning to synchronise with the baby's behaviour. Babies are individuals and have their own likes and dislikes and will communicate this through verbal and non-verbal signs.

If parents are encouraged to tune into their baby's cues they can be encouraged to develop their own special style of massage according to their baby's needs.

Below are some examples of the benefits of baby massage in practice ~ outline of successful Case Studies:

Case Study 1
Julia, Simon and Baby Drew

Background
Drew is Julia and Simons first child and is 3 months old. Julia had a natural birth, no complications and Drew weighed in at a healthy 7lb 8oz. Both Julia and Simon have admitted to being overawed and feeling slightly anxious with their new baby and were very keen to try baby massage to help with their own confidence in parenting and their bonding with Drew.

Session 1
Julia was instructed on the 5-minute routine and massaged the front of Drew's body and Simon did the routine on the back. Both found it very enjoyable, although a little awkward at first. Drew seem to enjoy it the most; he had been rather active prior to the massage but just lay there thoroughly mesmerised during the routine and then promptly fell into a deep relaxed sleep after a long drink.

Session 2—5 days later
On this occasion, Julia carried out the whole massage, whilst Simon watched. Both Simon and Julia had been practising their massage on Drew since the first session and commented on how enjoyable they were all finding it. Both sensed a more relaxed feeling and intimate bond between them and Drew, and also commented on better sleep patterns for the whole household. During this session Julia exhibited much more confidence when massaging Drew, who was now expressing his sheer enjoyment of his massage (by cooing, plenty of eye contact), particularly on his back. Again the massage proved acceptable to Drew as he fell into another deep sleep after a healthy feed from his bottle. At the end of this session both parents were shown gentle stretching techniques, which they would introduce into the routine over the next few days.

Session 3—3 days later
On this follow-up session, it was Simon who massaged Drew . . . with little instruction. Simon also incorporated some of the stretching techniques which they had been shown on the previous occasion. Little Drew responded very well to these as well, showing no resistance coupled with some smiling. It was very noticeable the increase in confidence which Simon showed, and the unconditional acceptance that Drew reciprocated to Simon. It was now just over a week since Julia and Simon had started massaging Drew with the benefits to all very clear. Both parents and child were showing much more bonding and also a sense of relaxation with each other.

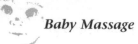

Outcomes

After just over a week of instruction sessions both Julia and Simon were very happy that they had started. On a personal level they felt much less tense and more confident in their parenting skills. They also commented that they were now able to get pretty much a good night's sleep, as they were massaging Drew before bedtime and finding that he was now sleeping through to around 6.45 am. Before they started massaging him, he would wake several times during the night. They will continue to massage Drew as they all enjoy it so much and the benefits that it has given them.

Case Study 2

Heather, John and Baby Amy

Background

Amy is Heather and John's second child. They already have one child, Peter, who is five. Since Amy was born, she has suffered very badly with colic, which has made her very restless and fretful. This is a new experience for Amy and John as they had no problems at all with Peter. They decided to try massage with Amy as a friend had told them about it and how it had helped with her baby who was very colicky. It was decided that Heather would attend the instruction sessions as it would be difficult for John due to his work schedules.

Session 1

The session took place at home in the lounge, which was fairly spacious. Both mum and baby were rather fractious as neither had had much sleep the previous night. Some soothing music was the first item of address to try to help relax mum and baby. Heather decided to use a large cushion to lay Amy on, so that she would be slightly inclined forward whilst the massage took place. Heather then sat with her back against the sofa with her legs astride and Amy in between them. Heather also decided to use some calendula oil for the massage as she already used a baby soap which was calendula based.

Initially, as the session commenced, Amy was not very receptive and tended to fidget. The massage was stopped and Heather picked Amy up to comfort her. When she had settled down, the massage was recommenced, but again Amy looked uncomfortable and this time began to cry. Heather picked her up to comfort her again and said that she didn't think Amy was going to respond and felt a bit disheartened.

After talking for a while and deciding to try again at a later date, the session was brought to a close to allow Mum and baby to try to get some much-needed sleep.

Some gentle touching strokes were suggested for Heather to try to familiarise Amy with before the next session.

Session 2—7 days later

Initially, Heather explained that she had persisted and tried some of the strokes with Amy who had gradually come to accept the stroking. This time Heather seemed more positive towards the session and Amy seemed less fretful. Both had also had a good night's sleep.

Heather again decided to use a large cushion to support Amy and sit with her back against the sofa. Soothing music was played and the massage commenced. During the initial strokes, Amy was a little fidgety but did start to relax and look at her mum as the massage continued. Heather followed the whole routine on the front and then turned Amy over onto her front to do her back at which point Amy started to cry. Heather picked her up to comfort her and then tried to lay her on her front again, but again Amy began to cry. It was then decided to try laying Amy on her left side, whilst Heather massaged her back.

Heather found this a little awkward at first but managed to adapt fairly quickly and Amy, although a little fidgety, did not cry. Heather concentrated on massaging Amy's back, which appeared to relax Amy until suddenly she began to fidget again. Amy began to get more agitated, when suddenly she burped quite loudly. As soon as this had happened she instantly relaxed again and remained relaxed whilst Heather massaged her back. This incident had an amusing effect, with Heather commenting that it was the first time that Amy had winded so loudly. The session was brought to a close with some gentle stretching to Amy's chest and arms.

Heather felt much more positive after this session and said that she would try longer sessions and more of the techniques with Amy before the next time.

Session 3—7 days later

The initial feedback from Heather was one of progress. Amy was now starting to respond well to the massage and was now even lying on her front. Heather also commented that she had been passing a lot more wind and seemed to be less fretful during the night.

Heather had been using the same positioning and location with Amy for the massages previous to this session, but decided to try massaging Amy on the bed this time, hoping she could do this nightly before Amy was put in her cot. Heather used a pillow for Amy to rest on whilst sitting with her back against the headboard and also decided to use very little oil as she personally was not to keen on using it. She also said that she had tried massaging Amy through her sleep suit and had found this much more convenient but with the same outcomes.

The session went very smoothly this time, with Amy watching her mum throughout the massage and appearing to be quite relaxed. At the end of the session, Heather did some gentle stretching with Amy and then picked her up to give her a feed. After Heather had fed Amy, she then massaged her back for quite some time, which really relaxed Amy and sent her into a restful sleep.

Outcomes

Heather continued with several more sessions until she felt confident to continue on her own. Each of the follow-up sessions was encouraging except for the fifth where Amy was very fretful. Heather commented that Amy had had a bad night prior to this session and was probably over tired.

Heather was pleased as Amy was now responding very well to the massage; she had also stopped using oil and was now massaging Amy through her sleep suit every night before settling her down. Amy was also showing encouraging signs and was less fretful, her sleep was less disturbed and she was also feeding better.

Case Study 3
Charlotte and baby Rhianna

Background

Charlotte is a single parent with two children, Harry who is 22 months and Rhianna who is 7 months. Rhianna has just started to crawl and is proving quite a challenge to Charlotte who has also been suffering with post-natal depression and finding two children very stressful.

Charlotte also admitted to feelings of guilt because she was finding it difficult to cope and was not bonding very well with Rhianna. She had heard about baby massage through her health visitor who had suggested she try as she felt it could possibly help Charlotte.

Session 1

The instruction took place at home. Charlotte lives in a small council flat with her two children and as the living room is fairly small she decided to try the massage in her bedroom. Charlotte thought it would be a good idea for Harry to sit and watch and maybe join in as it would be good for all of them and also keep Harry occupied during the session.

Charlotte had some music, which she already used to help her relax and decided to play this during the session. Charlotte positioned Rhianna on the bed and made her comfortable with some pillows; she knelt by the side of the bed and started the routine from there, using some baby lotion for the massage.

Both mum and baby seemed uncomfortable during the initial stages of the massage with Rhianna crying after a few minutes. Charlotte then sat up on the bed and picked up Rhianna and comforted her, whilst shedding a few tears herself. After a few minutes there was a certain empathy felt between them and Charlotte then gently placed Rhianna back down on the bed. This time Charlotte sat on the bed with her legs astride Rhianna and proceeded to follow the instruction this way. As the massage progressed Charlotte relaxed more, although Rhianna showed signs of uncertainty throughout and watched her mum with a strange frown.

Charlotte was able to massage Rhianna from start to finish, with little fuss from Rhianna throughout; she even did some gentle stretches to end the session. Charlotte commented that she was surprised how things had gone and even felt better after having a few tears to start with; she would try the routine with Rhianna over the next few days on a regular basis to see how things go. Charlotte was given plenty of aftercare advice to help her with Rhianna, particularly cuddles after the massages.

Session 2—5 days later
Charlotte said that she had continued with the massages since the last time and that Rhianna had been watching her less intently each time. She had also included Harry during the sessions as she felt it had also calmed him down a bit as well. She was still feeling very low herself but admitted that she had felt slightly better when she did the massage.

This session was again in the bedroom, but with Charlotte starting in a closer position to Rhianna. Harry was sleeping so didn't take part this time. During the massage there was a noticeable difference in Rhianna and also Charlotte herself. Rhianna showed signs of being more accepting of her mother's touch and was less tense, which showed in her body language and eyes. Charlotte was more relaxed as well and there were several smiles exchanged between Mum and baby during the massage.

After the massage, Charlotte sat and held Rhianna whilst she drank some water and talked to her very lovingly. She commented that she felt happy at the way Rhianna seemed more relaxed in her presence and showed signs of pleasure by having the massage.

Session 3—5 days later
Charlotte had continued with the massage and even though Rhianna was now starting to crawl had found that she was willing for her mum to give her a regular massage. Charlotte said that it was helping her and that she was feeling fewer of the guilt feelings she had experienced previously. She was also beginning to feel

slightly less overwhelmed as she felt that she was beginning to enjoy her daughter's company rather than it being a burden. It was also having a knock-on effect on Harry too as he was joining in most of the sessions and being helpful rather than a hindrance.

This session was enjoyed by all the family with Harry, as best he could, helping Charlotte to prepare for the massage. Harry also had a little go himself which Rhianna didn't seem to mind. The session ended with the family having a lovely cuddle together and sharing a drink of water. After the cuddle and drink of water, both Harry and Rhianna settled down for a sleep. Charlotte expressed that she still felt low but that the massage was definitely helping her. She did feel closer to her daughter and son and that in itself gave her a lift. She was very keen to continue with the guided session and would continue the massage on her own.

Outcomes
The instruction sessions continued for a couple of months on a regular basis, with Charlotte continuing the massage alone in between the sessions and then afterwards.

Charlotte has said that she found it very beneficial as it had certainly helped her to bond better with Rhianna and whilst it was not an instant cure-all for the way she had been feeling it had definitely helped to lift her spirits, particularly whilst giving the massage. She also commented that she had definitely been dwelling less on the way she was feeling and becoming more occupied with her daughter's development.

Questions for Review

1. i) List six physiological benefits of baby massage for babies

_____
_____
_____
_____
_____
_____

   ii) List four psychological benefits of baby massage for babies

_____
_____
_____
_____

   iii) Describe four benefits of baby massage for parents

_____
_____
_____
_____

2. Describe the role of baby massage as an important form of communication

_____
_____
_____
_____
_____
_____

03 An Introduction to Pregnancy Massage

Pregnancy is a special time in a woman's life and it is therefore important for expectant mums to feel nurtured as they prepare themselves for the birth of their baby. During pregnancy women may experience a variety of physical ailments and problems including backache, swollen ankles, aching muscles, fatigue, breast soreness, heartburn to name but a few. In addition there are the psychological effects of the pregnancy which include increased feelings of stress, concerns about the baby's health, change of body image and coping with the challenges of motherhood.

Massage during pregnancy requires certain adaptations in terms of positioning and pressure in order to work safely and effectively, however actual use of techniques are largely the same as for non-pregnant clients.

This chapter offers an introduction to how massage can be used to relieve tension during pregnancy, including techniques to ease back strain, and reduce fluid retention, whilst helping to balance the emotions during this important time. Massage during pregnancy can also help to prepare expectant mothers for labour and make the post-natal period less stressful.

By the end of this chapter you will be able to relate the following knowledge to your role as instructor/carer/parent:

❋ The benefits of massage during pregnancy
❋ Safety precautions and recommendations
❋ The safe use of essential oils during pregnancy
❋ Comfortable positioning for massage during pregnancy
❋ Practical techniques for common minor problems during pregnancy
❋ Stretching and relaxation techniques during pregnancy
❋ Post-natal massage care.

The Benefits of Massage during Pregnancy

During pregnancy, a woman's body undergoes a great many changes in preparation for childbirth. The changes in a woman's body, coupled with the natural anxieties associated with pregnancy, can all be stress-inducing.

Massage can be of great benefit in helping expectant mothers to prepare themselves physically and emotionally for childbirth and motherhood.

Pregnancy massage is therefore the ideal foundation to baby massage.

Massage during Pregnancy can help to:

* increase the circulation of blood to all areas of the body (including the placenta), thereby bringing greater nutrition to the tissues and enhancing removal of waste
* reduce strain on the muscles of the lower back, abdomen and shoulders
* increase the tone of muscles that have become weakened and strained during pregnancy
* improve the elasticity of the skin
* encourage rest and relaxation that is much needed during pregnancy
* reduce fatigue due to increased oxygen absorption into the tissues, and waste products being more readily eliminated
* stabilise hormonal levels through increased stimulation of glandular secretions
* increase energy levels
* elevate the mood due to the increased production of endorphins (whatever the expectant mother feels is passed on to her baby)
* reduce fluid retention due to the increased and more efficient circulation of lymph
* soothe nerves and promote relaxation through sedation of the nervous system
* prepare the body for a more comfortable pregnancy
* enable mother and expectant father to communicate lovingly with their baby.

Contra-indications to Massage during Pregnancy

There are certain instances in which it is not advisable to receive a massage during pregnancy. These include:

* during the first trimester of pregnancy
* if there is a decrease in fetal movement over a 24-hour period
* if suffering from a fever
* a severe headache
* if you have an infection
* if experiencing morning sickness, vomiting or nausea
* vaginal bleeding or discharge
* faintness
* pain in the abdomen, or anywhere else in the body
* excessive swelling to the extremities
* immediately after eating (it is best to wait one and a half to two hours).

NB. It is important to seek advice from your GP before receiving massage if you suffer from a medical condition, or have any complications with your pregnancy.

Adaptations for Massage during Pregnancy

The main consideration when massaging a pregnant client is comfortable positioning. During the second and third trimester the client will usually receive massage in the supine or side-lying position, alternatively they may be seated in a chair. It is important for the therapist to discuss the best positioning with the client for ease of comfort and to experiment with different ways.

Care should be taken to offer plenty of support to the chest and lower abdominal area, as well as the ankles and knees. If ankles are swollen, it is helpful to elevate the knees and the feet using bolsters while supine, so that the feet are higher than the knees.

NB. Deep abdominal massage should be avoided during pregnancy, and pressure strokes in general should be soothing and relaxing.

Comfortable positions for Massage during Pregnancy

Side-lying posture

This is one of the most comfortable positions during pregnancy, particularly as the pregnancy progresses. The mother lies on one side, with the top leg bent at the hip and knee. A pillow is placed under the bent knee, and one is given to rest her arm on and one to hug against her chest.

One side of the back and hip may be massaged in this position and then the client may move to lie on the other side in order to get both sides of the back and hip massaged.

Side lying position during pregnancy showing kneading around the scapula with the fingers/ thumbs ▼

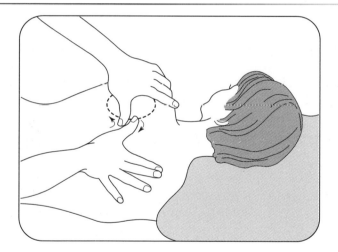

Seated massage

Some clients prefer to be seated in a chair for massage. The mother sits astride a comfortable chair and leans into the backrest, with a pillow(s) for support in the chest and abdominal area.

Considerations for the therapist are to select a chair that is at a sufficient height for them to carry out massage to the upper back without straining. It is preferable for the therapist to stand whilst carrying out massage to the upper back, but usually it is better to sit behind the client when massaging the lower back.

Seated position for pregnancy massage to the upper back showing kneading down either side of the spine with the thumbs ▼

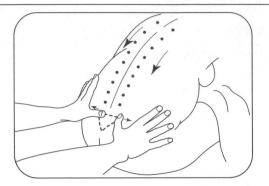

Seated position for pregnancy massage to the lower back showing massaging the heel of the hand into the base of the spine ▼

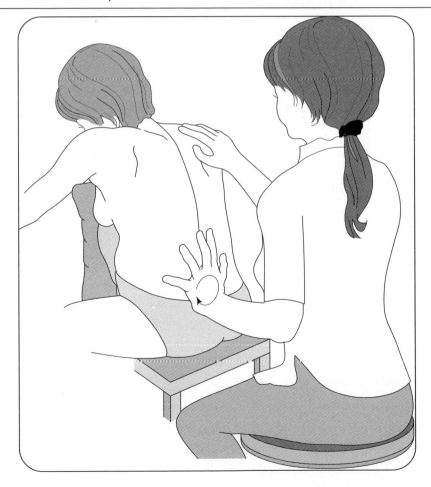

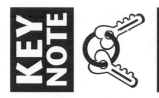

When massaging a pregnant client, therapists may find it helpful to use a chair that is especially designed for seated massage, which is both comfortable and adjustable.

Supine

As the uterus presses on the large abdominal vein (vena cava) when the mother lies on her back, the massage is more comfortably carried out when the headrest of a couch is semi-reclined and with plenty of supports under the head, upper back, knees and ankles. Some clients may be more comfortable sat upright in a chair with their legs elevated.

Prone

Some clients may be happy to lie prone until the later stages of their pregnancy, in which case there will need to be careful placements of supports to facilitate comfort. Some companies produce body cushions/supports specifically designed for this purpose. (Refer to resource section, Physique Management Company.)

Prone position using massage supports ▼

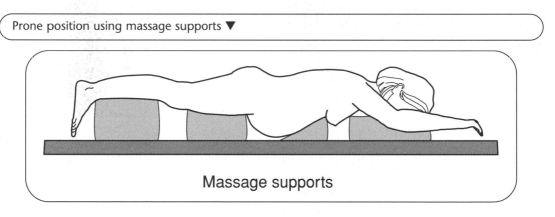

Massage supports

Pregnancy Massage Oils

There are a variety of different massage oils that may be used during pregnancy, although it is preferable to use a medium that is more nourishing to the skin such as jojoba, olive, grapeseed or coconut, for example.

There are a number of specially blended pure oils on the market for pregnant women (see Resource section for details on Neals Yard Remedies who sell a Mother's Massage Oil). Some women may prefer the use of a cream rich in vitamin E to help improve the elasticity of the skin.

The Safe Use of Essential Oils during Pregnancy

When considering the use of essential oils in pregnancy massage it is important to remember that as they are absorbed into the bloodstream and can cross the placental barrier, they may have the potential to affect the foetus. There are important considerations when proposing to use essential oils in pregnancy massage as follows.

Important Advice for Baby Massage Instructors

❋ Avoid blending essential oils for use in pregnancy massage if you are not qualified and insured to practise aromatherapy professionally—use a pure blend of oils from a reputable supplier.

❋ If you are qualified to use essential oils, research known safety data to avoid potentially toxic essential oils that may be harmful to mother and foetus.

❋ Always use essential oils in a lower dilution during pregnancy (in 20ml of carrier/base oil you would add a total combination of *up to* 4–5 drops of essential oils).

Important Advice for the Pregnant Woman

❋ Avoid using any essential oils during the first trimester of pregnancy.

❋ Seek advice from a qualified aromatherapist before using essential oils during pregnancy.

❋ If the pregnancy is uncomplicated and is progressing well, essential oils should be used in a much lower proportion than normal.

❋ Always buy essential oils from a reputable supplier who can give correct advice on their safe use during pregnancy (see Resource section for Neals Yard Remedies).

Common examples of essential oils which should be avoided during pregnancy include:

Basil, Clary Sage, Fennel, Juniper, Marjoram, Nutmeg, Rosemary and Thyme

Examples of toxic oils to be avoided in aromatherapy (including use during pregnancy) include:

Aniseed, Arnica, Mugwort, Pennroyal, Sassafras, Savory, Thuja, Wintergreen and Wormwood.

Essential oils which are considered safe, when used in the correct proportions, for use in pregnancy (after the first trimester) include:

Bergamot, Chamomile (Roman), Grapefruit, Lavender, Lemon, Lime, Mandarin, Neroli, Orange (sweet), Petitgrain, Rose, Sandalwood, Tangerine, Ylang Ylang

Essential oils which are considered to be useful during labour include:

Chamomile (Roman), Clary Sage, Geranium, Frankincense, Jasmin, Lavender

Essential oils useful for the post-natal period include:

Bergamot, Cypress, Frankincense, Geranium, Jasmine, Juniper, Lavender, Patchouli and Rose

Practical Techniques for Common Minor Problems during Pregnancy

Backache

During pregnancy the ligaments around the lower back and hip become softer and stretch in preparation for labour. This can put excess strain on the lower back and pelvis and can cause the discomfort of backache. As the baby increases in size, it causes the hollow in the lower back (lumbar curve) to increase and this, along with the added weight gain, contributes to backache.

Practical Massage Techniques to help ease Backache during Pregnancy

The following techniques may be demonstrated with the therapist standing behind the client:

1 Perform long sweeping (effleurage) strokes up either side of the spine with full contact of the hands, and return back down with a lighter stroke. Repeat × 6.

2 Support one side of the mother's upper back with your hand and perform large overlapping circles either side of the spine (away from the spine) with the palmar surface of the hand. Repeat × 3.

Large overlapping circles either side of the spine with the palmar surface of the hand ▼

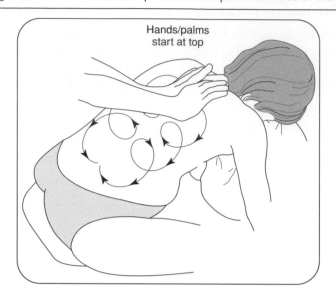

Hands/palms
start at top

3 Repeat on the other side.

4 Knead the muscles at the top of the shoulders with both hands.

5 Squeeze the muscles at the top of the shoulder between the fingers and the heel of your hands, extend the techniques down the upper arms.

6 Knead around the scapula with the fingers/thumbs, concentrating on easing out any knots of tension. Repeat the other side.

7 Knead down either side of the spine with the thumbs. Repeat × 6.

The following techniques may be demonstrated with the therapist sitting behind the client.

1 Support one side of the hip and turn to the opposite side of the client's lower back and circle around the back of the hip with the palmar surface of the hand. Repeat × 6.

2 Now, facing the client's lower back slide with both thumbs from the lower back and across the back of the hip. Repeat × 3.

3 Thumb knead around the sacrum and the back of the hip with both hands × 3.

Thumb knead around the sacrum and the back of the hip ▼

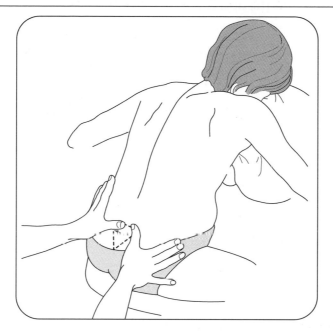

4 Slowly and gently massage the heel of the hand into the base of the spine × 6.

Most of the above techniques may be adapted for use when the client is lying on her side, with the obvious difference being that one side of the back and hip is massaged at a time.

Stretches to help ease Backache during Pregnancy

The following stretches are best carried out on the floor supported by a soft mat or pillows.

1 Knees to Chest Stretch

✱ The mother lies on the floor, with knees bent and whilst breathing in brings one knee slowly towards the chest.

✱ Upon breathing out the leg is then slowly straightened back onto the floor.

✱ This is then repeated with the other leg.

✱ Then both knees are brought up towards the chest and a gentle rocking movement is performed in a circular motion (clockwise and anticlockwise) which helps to give the lower back (sacrum) a gentle massage.

2 Knee to Chest Twist

✱ The mother lies on the floor and slowly pulls both knees towards the chest.

✻ The bent knees are then dropped over to one side and the head is turned in the opposite direction and the arm is raised above the head.

Knee to Chest Twist ▼

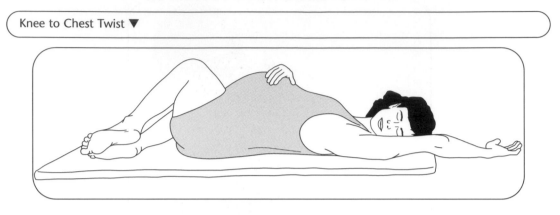

Constipation and Flatulence

Constipation and flatulence are very common problems during pregnancy. The high levels of progesterone at this time cause relaxation of the smooth muscles of the bowel and reduce intestinal activity. The pressure from the developing baby pressing on the intestines also inhibits normal bowel activity.

The pressure can feel uncomfortable, but massage and relaxation exercises that relax and strengthen the abdominal muscles will help to ease the discomfort. Intestinal gas builds up as the waste products remain in the intestines without being eliminated.

Practical Techniques to help ease Constipation and Flatulence during Pregnancy

It is not advisable to carry out deep abdominal pressure during pregnancy; however, the following techniques are very beneficial for constipation and flatulence.

1 Gentle rhythmic massage over the abdomen in a clockwise direction with alternate hands (one hand performs half of the circle and the other hand completes it). Repeat × 6.

Massage over the abdomen in a clockwise direction with alternate hands ▼

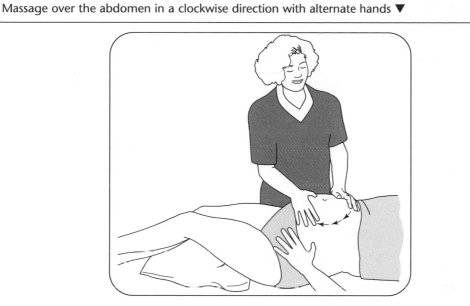

2   Lifting up and down the sides of the abdomen; both hands start either side of the abdomen and then gently pull up towards the centre and then back down. Repeat × 3.

Lifting up and down the sides of the abdomen ▼

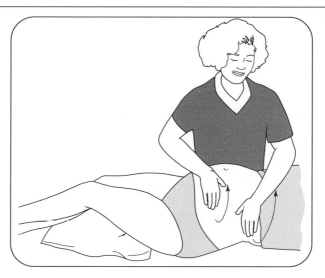

3   Gentle stroking with both hands from the centre of the abdomen across to the sides of the waist and sliding round towards the back. Gently lift from the back up the sides of the waist as you reverse the stroke. Repeat × 6.

Gentle stroking to the sides of the waist and back ▼

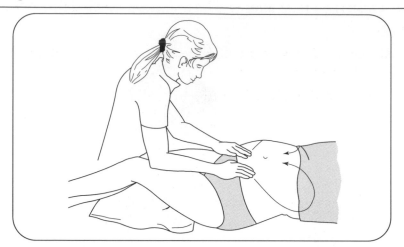

Stretching Techniques for Relieving Abdominal Pressure

These techniques are best performed lying on the floor on a supportive mat or pillows.

1   Pelvic Tilt

❋ The mother lies on the floor, with knees bent and feet pulled up towards the buttocks (arms rest at the sides of the body).

❋ Slowly lift the pelvis to maximum tilt, whilst keeping the feet on the floor.

❋ Hold for 5 to 10 seconds.

❋ Slowly return to the original position by lowering the upper back first and slowly down the rest of the spine.

Pelvic Tilt ▼

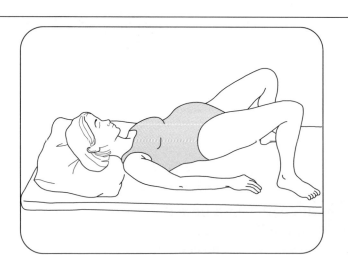

2   Cat Stretch

❋ The mother kneels on the hands and knees, whilst keeping the back straight.

❋ Then inhales.

❋ Upon exhalation the lower back is rounded out, by bringing the chin to the chest. Hold to a count of 5.

❋ Inhale and return to the original position.

Cat Stretch ▼

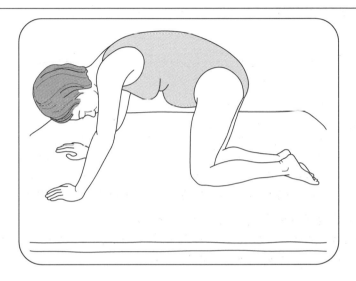

3   Pose of the Child Stretch

❋ The mother kneels on the floor with legs slightly spread apart, bends forward and places head to one side on a cushion on the floor.

❋ Both arms are brought in close to the body and rest alongside the legs.

❋ Stay in this position for about one minute and then turn the head to the other side and repeat.

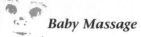
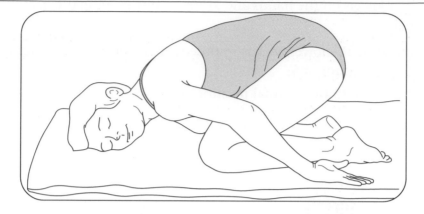

Pose of the Child Stretch ▼

Fatigue

Fatigue is a very common problem in pregnancy as even when the body is at rest, it is working harder than it ever did before the pregnancy. During the first trimester, tiredness tends to be worse as the body is working very hard to produce the placenta, which will provide the baby's life support system.

Women will feel tired during pregnancy due to the fact that their metabolism slows down, hormonal changes occur, blood volume increases slowing down circulation and excess weight is being carried.

Oedema

Excess accumulation of fluid in the extremities is a common complaint, particularly in the later stages of pregnancy. Pregnant women commonly suffer with swollen ankles and this is usually as a result of fetal head pressure on the pelvic veins, which restricts the blood flow from the legs, along with the excess weight.

Practical Techniques to help ease Fatigue and Oedema

The most effective techniques to help ease fatigue during pregnancy are to the legs and feet. The techniques to the back are also useful at relieving fatigue as they help to improve the mother's posture (poor postural movements utilise more energy than is needed for proper body alignment).

Pregnancy Massage Techniques for the Legs and Feet

The client is ideally positioned in a seated or semi-reclined position, with props/supports under the knees and ankles.

1   Start by using long continuous sweeping (effleurage) strokes with both hands from the ankle up to the top of the thighs (returning back down to the ankles with a lighter stroke). Repeat × 6.

2   Now work from just above the knee up to the top of the hip, gradually increasing the pressure on the upward stroke (returning to above the knee with a lighter stroke). Repeat × 6.

Effleurage from above the knee up to the top of the hip ▼

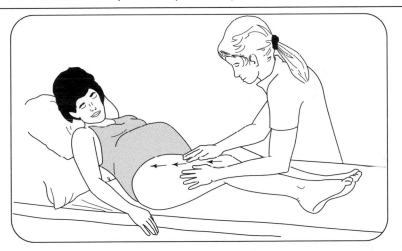

3   Support one side of the thigh with one hand and use overlapping circular movements with the palmar surface of the hand, gradually working up one side of the leg and returning down towards the knee with a long continuous stroke. Repeat × 3 each side.

Overlapping circular movements with the palmar surface of the hand to the thigh ▼

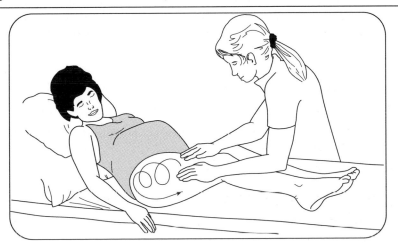

4 Shape the thumb and fingers of both hands into a tunnel shape and with one placed in front of the other slide up from above the knee towards the hip and return down the side of the thigh with a lighter stroke. Repeat × 6 progressively increasing in pressure.

Tunnelling movement to the thighs ▼

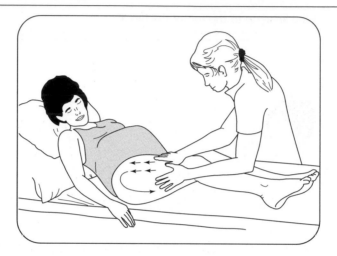

Without breaking contact stroke down the ankles.

5 Lightly stroke around the inside and outside of the ankle bones, with pads of fingers of both hands in a circular movement. Repeat × 3.

Stroking around the inside and outside of the ankle bones ▼

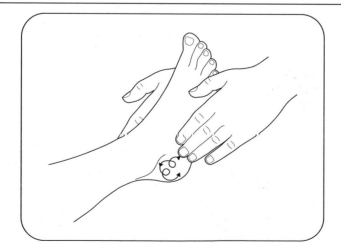

6 Massage around the front of the ankles with pads of both fingers in a circular motion, concentrating on the important area of the ankle to help alleviate hip pain in pregnancy. Repeat several times (see illustration).

Kneading the front of the ankle (important area for hip/back pain) ▼

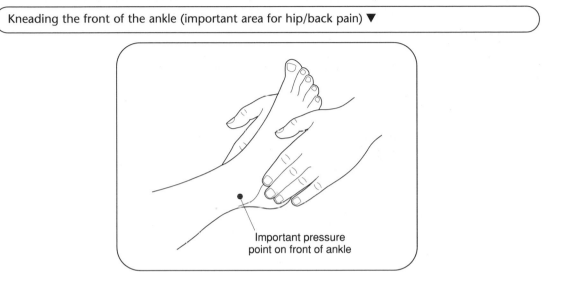

Important pressure point on front of ankle

7 Lift the leg a few inches and cup the hands under the heel. Slide the other hand along the Achilles' tendon working towards you. Alternate with the left hand in a flowing motion. Repeat several times.

Lift and stretching to the Achilles tendon ▼

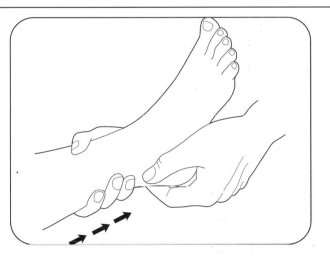

8 Support under the ankle with one hand and rotate the ankle joint in a clockwise and anticlockwise direction. Repeat × 3 each way.

9 Placing both thumbs of the top of the feet, below the toes, with index fingers placed on the sole of the feet, stroke downwards towards the ankle with the emphasis of the pressure being on the thumbs on the top of the feet. The pressure upwards back towards the toes should be on the sole of the feet with the index fingers. Repeat this several times, progressively increasing in pressure.

Drainage movement to the feet with the thumb and index finger ▼

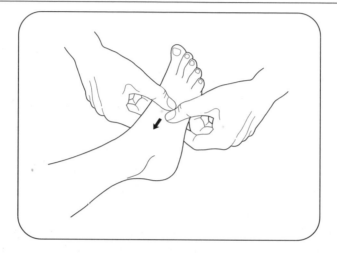

10 Turn slightly to the side to knead in a circular motion down the inner arch of the foot with alternate thumbs. Repeat × 3.

11 Massage the fist of one hand into the sole of the foot, whilst supporting the top of the foot with the other hand. Repeat × 3.

12 Conclude by stroking with both hands from foot to ankle, with pressure on the downwards stroke. Repeat × 6 progressively lightening the pressure.

NB. It is preferable if the client can rest in a position with her limbs elevated for a while after the massage to assist drainage and absorption of fluid. At this point the client may want to turn on her side, which is the posture that provides the most efficient venous blood return (particularly the left side).

Stretching Techniques to help Fatigue and Oedema

Lying with the feet up the side of the wall and hold there whilst performing several deep breaths in and out.

Headaches

Headaches during pregnancy are commonly caused by hormonal changes; however there are other contributory factors such as fatigue, tension, sinus congestion, emotional stress and hunger.

The techniques illustrated on pages 26–27 are all effective for stress-related headaches; areas to concentrate on would be the neck, shoulders and back. Some pregnant clients find their headache is relieved after a good foot massage.

Other Considerations when carrying out Pregnancy Massage

Besides the obvious difference in positioning for maximum comfort, there are several other considerations:

❋ Pregnant women generally feel hotter during pregnancy due to an increased blood supply to the skin, and therefore the temperature of the room/number of coverings may need to be adjusted (it is advisable to have some cool water to hand).

❋ The skin may be more sensitive due to the increased blood supply; care may need to be taken in the choice of massage medium (some women experience itchiness during pregnancy).

❋ Pregnant women will pass water more frequently due to the increased pressure on the bladder, and as massage will increase the flow of urine, it is therefore best for the client to visit the toilet before the treatment commences.

❋ Certain smells may make women feel nauseous during pregnancy; care will therefore need to be taken in the choice of medium and essential oils (if applicable).

❋ As tiredness is a common side effect of pregnancy, the pregnant client may become uncomfortable or intolerant of an extended massage (it is best therefore to limit the massage to shorter more frequent sessions).

❋ Feeling faint is more common in pregnancy because of hormonal changes taking place in the body. It is more likely to happen when getting up too quickly from lying down on the back (it is therefore usually more comfortable for pregnant women to lie on their side).

❋ Pregnant clients may need to change position more frequently during massage (always be ready with supports and suggestions for improving comfort).

Post-natal Massage Care

The post-natal period is an important recovery time when the uterus returns to its pre-pregnancy size and hormonal levels become re-established. Fatigue, depression, after pains, breast soreness, general stiffness and soreness after labour are all common symptoms experienced after childbirth.

A considerable amount of energy goes into looking after a baby and therefore of equal importance is post-natal care of the self, paying attention in particular to adequate rest, proper nutrition, plenty of fluids and emotional support, all of which can help speed up recovery.

Massage plays an important role (after the post-natal health check) and can help mothers to feel nurtured after the physical and emotional demands of childbirth.

Post-natal Depression

During the first few weeks after childbirth, most women experience what is often referred to as the 'baby blues'. Symptoms include feeling emotional, irrational, irritable, anxious and weepy, often bursting into tears for no apparent reason.

The cause is the change in the hormone levels experienced after delivery of the baby. Throughout pregnancy, the hormone levels rise to accommodate the growing baby and by the time the labour commences, the levels of progesterone and oestrogen are 50 per cent higher than they were before the pregnancy. After childbirth, the levels of these hormones fall suddenly and dramatically, so much so that within a matter of hours they are below the levels they were before the pregnancy began.

The symptoms associated with the baby blues usually only last for a few days. If the baby blues seem to be getting worse and the symptoms become more distressing post-natal depression could be starting to develop. Post-natal depression is not always easy to recognise as a baby's arrival changes everything and it is easy for new mums to blame their symptoms on all the new demands on their time and energy.

Post-natal depression is thought to affect at least one in ten women. It usually occurs two to eight weeks after delivery, although in some cases the depression can appear up to six months or even a year after the birth of the baby.

With post-natal depression the following symptoms may apply:

✽ inability to stop crying
✽ feeling of hopelessness

* feeling permanently tired and lethargic
* simple household tasks seem too much effort
* feeling generally unwell
* suffering from head, back or neck pain
* feeling anxious
* inability to relax
* sleeping badly
* memory loss or inability to concentrate
* inability to cope with meeting people or answering the door
* experiencing panic and confusion in everyday situations
* loss of interest in looking after self or baby.

It is extremely important that mothers suffering from post-natal depression receive support from their families and they are advised to seek help and support from their health visitor and GP.

There are several associations who may be contacted for much needed support with post-natal depression. See Resource section at the back of this book. Massage can also provide a supportive role for the post-natal period as it can help women to feel nurtured and cared for, whilst helping them back to an emotional and physical state of balance.

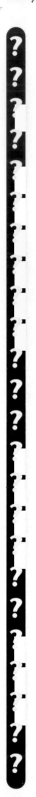

Questions for Review

1. State five benefits of a woman receiving massage during pregnancy

    _____
    _____
    _____
    _____
    _____
    _____
    _____

2. List six examples when it is not considered safe for a woman to receive massage during pregnancy

    _____
    _____
    _____
    _____
    _____
    _____
    _____
    _____
    _____
    _____

3. What is one of the most comfortable positions for massage during the later stages of pregnancy and why?

    _____
    _____
    _____
    _____
    _____

4. State two other important considerations when carrying out pregnancy massage, other than positioning

    _____

    _____

    _____

5. State three important safety precautions associated with the use of essential oils for pregnant women

    _____

    _____

    _____

04 Baby Anatomy & Physiology

Baby Anatomy & Physiology

Physiologically a baby's growth pattern is not complete until about the age of three. The visible changes in the size of a baby as it develops are as a result of changes in bone, muscles and fat.

This chapter aims to provide a comprehensive insight into a baby's anatomy and physiology, which will be of mutual interest to instructors and parents alike. Although anatomy and physiology is generally a uniform subject, there are a number of significant differences in the anatomy and physiology of babies in relation to adults, all of which are explored in this chapter.

The differences in anatomy will help instructors and parents to understand the ways in which massaging babies is distinctly different from massaging adults.

By the end of this chapter, you will be able to relate the following knowledge in relation to anatomy and physiology of babies to your role as an instructor or parent/carer:

* Skeletal Development
* Development of Teeth
* Muscular Development
* Baby's Skin and Tissues
* Neural Development
* The Cardiovascular System
* The Digestive System
* The Renal System
* The Respiratory System
* The Reproductive System
* The Immune System.

Skeletal Development in Babies

A baby's skeletal development changes and develops according to age, genetics, hormones, individual muscular development and the forces exerted upon it by parts of the musculo-skeletal system.

Development proceeds from the top to the bottom, following the *cephalocaudal* law of growth.

As babies' heads develop first, it explains why their heads look out of proportion to the bodies in the first year of their life. Development also proceeds from the inner parts to the extremities, following the *proximodistal* law of growth. This explains why babies' hands and feet look small in relation to their bodies.

Proximodistal/cephalocaudal law of growth ▼

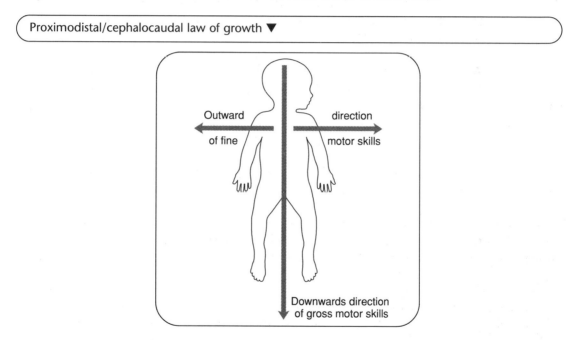

It is interesting to note that a baby's head at birth accounts for around 25 per cent of the length of the entire body and almost 33 per cent of the body's weight, whilst the arms and the legs make up only 8–16 per cent.

At birth most of a baby's skeleton is composed of bone, but some parts such as the arms, legs, hand and foot bones are made up of cartilage and do not turn into bone (by a process called ossification) until late adolescence. The cartilage continues to grow before ossifying, which allows the rapid growth of childhood to occur.

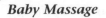

Baby's skeleton illustrating incomplete ossification ▼

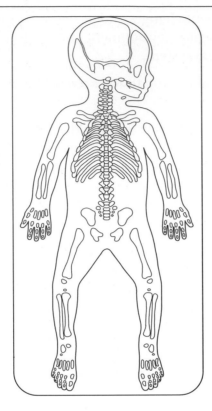

The bones of a new-born baby are soft, which is one of the reasons why they appear very floppy but is also the reason why later they are supple enough to put their feet in their mouth!

A new-born baby may have as many as 300 distinct bones, but many of these fuse together as the child grows (the average number of bones in an adult is 206). During the first year of a baby's life the bones increase in number, as well as size and weight. The wrist bones, for example are not present at birth, but by the time a baby reaches 12 months he has three. As the bones develop the baby will acquire greater control of hand and wrist movements which enables him to hold things more securely.

In a new-born the entire vertebral column is a concave forward shape forming the primary curves present at birth (thoracic and sacral). When the infant begins to assume an erect posture, secondary curves, which are convex, form. For example, the cervical curve appears when an infant begins to hold the head up at around 3 months of age; the lumbar curve appears when the baby begins to walk.

Changes in a baby's posture are related to the development of the secondary spinal curves. At 3 to 4 months, babies pull their heads up and try to balance the head on top of the spine to fix gaze. At 8 months they have the strength to sit up and the lumbar curve is evident. At one year a baby exhibits a wide gait in order to stand against gravity and balance a heavy skull. This may cause the lumbar curve to be exaggerated and the abdomen to protrude, as the baby tries to hold the upper part of the body erect until the back muscles develop the strength to maintain posture.

At birth, the bones in a baby's skull are not fully ossified and are joined by flexible bands of fibrous tissues called fontanelles, to enable rapid growth of the brain during the first few years of life. The anterior fontanelles can be felt in the midline of the skull above the brow, and close gradually in the first 18 months of life, whereas the smaller posterior fontanelle, found towards the back of the baby's head in the midline, is normally closed by six weeks.

The normal fontanelle is flat but may pulsate with the heart beat or bulge when the baby coughs or strains. It may feel soft or slightly springy from the support of the layer of cerebral spinal fluid, which circulates to cushion and protect the brain.

The fontanelles ▼

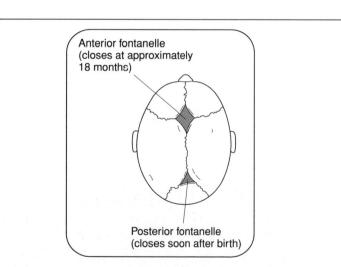

Anterior fontanelle
(closes at approximately
18 months)

Posterior fontanelle
(closes soon after birth)

By the time a child is two years of age the skull bones will have fused together. The facial bones on a baby are only very small; the jaw is small at birth, with usually no teeth apparent.

Babies and small children have small facial sinuses which make them subject to a lot of infections and runny noses, as infections become lodged in the crevices.

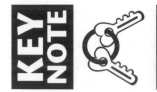

KEY NOTE

Babies' bones are softer with higher water content than adults' and therefore care must be taken to avoid applying too much pressure during massage, which may cause discomfort and injury.

Teeth

There is usually a wide variation in the development of babies' teeth, although they usually come through in the same order. Teeth may be present in the newborn, but generally they start to erupt at around 6 to 8 months. Generally the first teeth to develop are the lower central incisors which come through at around 6 months. These are usually followed by the upper central incisors at between 6 to 8 months.

At around 9 months, the four lateral incisors then appear on either side of the central incisors. These are followed by the four front molars at between ten and fourteen months.

Between 16 and 18 months the canines develop to fill the gap between the lateral incisors and the front molars. The back molars do not appear until around the end of the second year.

By two-and-a-half years most children have all 20 of their baby (or milk) teeth, as opposed to 32 permanent teeth which will start to appear at around six years of age.

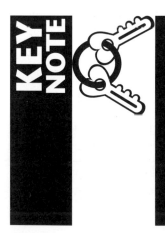

KEY NOTE

Teething starts long before a baby's teeth start to appear, which can be anytime between three and twelve months. Signs of teething include increased salivation, red gums, a raised temperature, a cough, red cheeks, loose stools and ammoniacal nappy rash. Babies will often appear fretful, distressed or irritable when teething due to the pain and discomfort experienced.

This is an ideal time for a parent to employ some non-invasive massage strokes to the hands and feet to give comfort and help to alleviate pain through the release of endorphins.

Muscular Development in Babies

A baby's muscle fibres are virtually all present at birth. Like babies' bones, their muscles fibres are initially small and watery, becoming larger and thicker later in childhood.

Although a baby can move quite vigorously at birth, their muscles are not fully developed and will grow in length and breadth and thicken as the baby develops.

Muscles grow rapidly during infancy and in the first 18 months the muscle mass increases twice as fast as the mass of bones. The number of muscle fibres does not increase (a baby has the same number of muscle fibres at birth as he will as an adult) but the fibres become longer and thicker. Babies' muscles develop from the inside out and from the head down.

In early infancy, most of a baby's muscle power is required for breathing and therefore the respiratory muscles of a young baby are twice the size of the muscles in the arms. This explains why a young baby's arms are so small in proportion to their chests.

As the limbs become more active, the muscles of the arms and legs grow faster. The earliest sign of controlled muscle movement is a baby's control of the neck muscles which lift the head. By three months a baby's neck and back muscle may be strong enough for him to raise his head and chest. By around 6 months, a baby may be able to sit alone momentarily and by 8 months may be strong enough to sit up unsupported for a while. The next stage, once the muscles of the legs have developed, is to stand and then walk.

The most important factors affecting muscle development include hormones present in the body, physical activity and diet.

The more physical activity a baby has, the more strength and co-ordination they will have with their motor development. A new-born baby does not have enough muscle strength or control to support its head, but as the muscles start to develop they provide a basis for future development of gross motor skills such as walking.

Some muscles take a long time to gain strength and size, in order that they may be brought under control (for instance a baby's leg muscles).

Massage can be of great benefit in encouraging muscular co-ordination and joint mobility in babies.

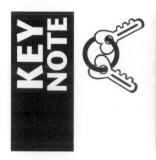

KEY NOTE

As a baby's muscles comprise only a quarter of their total body weight and are underdeveloped initially, it is important to avoid applying too much pressure when massaging, by using mainly the middle and ring fingers to apply the massage strokes in the early stages, before establishing more contact with the palmar surface of the hand as the baby grows in size.

Baby's Skin

The skin is an important sensory organ to a baby, as it is through the skin that a baby receives many messages from the outside world, particularly those of temperature and human touch.

A new-born baby's skin is thin, but the nerve endings are as numerous and as well developed (although, of course, not as large) as an adult's.

The sensory area of the brain (the sensory cortex), where the messages of sensory nerves are processed, is more mature than any other sensory area of the brain. This means that the new-born's skin has acute skin sensation and is therefore extremely sensitive to touch, being able to feel the slightest of touch.

As touch is an important part of a baby's physical and emotional growth, massaging is a natural way of a parent's inclination to cuddle and caress their baby.

Another important function of the skin is to control temperature. Young babies cannot control their temperature through the skin as effectively as older babies, children and adults. Therefore, it is important to keep the baby in a constant warm temperature and keep them warmly wrapped to avoid cooling down too much.

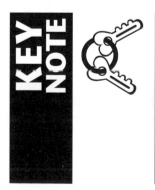

KEY NOTE

The skin tells us through its numerous sensory nerve endings, whether sensations are pleasurable or painful.

It is important to stress to parents the importance of the amount of pressure applied to skin when massaging their baby. For instance, in a new-born, gentle stroking is appropriate whereas once that skin is more developed and tissue density has increased gentle petrissage may be applied.

Adipose tissue

The composition of a baby's tissues is initially made up of a high proportion of fat (known as adipose tissue) which is designed as a protective layer and is important in temperature control of the new-born.

The subcutaneous fat, which is laid down at approximately 34 weeks prenatally, will eventually disappear as the child develops.

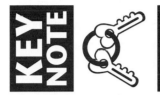

KEY NOTE

Although babies have a high proportion of fat which generates heat, they will lose heat very quickly so it is essential that the room in which the massage instruction takes place is maintained at a warm temperature.

Neural Development in Babies

The growth and development of the central nervous system is remarkable during the early childhood years. Neural development occurs at several stages during childhood, although the anatomy of a baby's brain is remarkably complete at birth.

The brain has many different functions, including controlling heart rate, respiration, body temperature and appetite, receiving and interpreting touch, visual and sound stimuli, controlling body posture, movement and thinking.

At birth, some parts of the brain are already functioning well, such as those that control attention, absorbing new information and basic baby activities of sleeping, waking, feeding and eliminating waste through the bowel and bladder. However, the parts of the brain that control the more complex activities such as controlled movement, language, understanding and thinking, continue to develop after birth and are almost, but not altogether complete by the time a child is two.

A baby's brain is approximately 33 per cent of its adult size at birth, but only 25 per cent of its eventual weight. In the new-born, the brain is 10–12 per cent of a baby's body weight and doubles in the first year of life. At birth, the head circumference is in excess of the chest circumference by around 2–3cm, however, at between one to two years the head circumference equals that of the chest.

By the age of one, a baby's brain will have reached 66 per cent of its adult weight and by five or six years of age this figure increases to 90 per cent. (The brain continues to grow and increase in size for the next 20 years, or so.)

The principal cells of the brain are neurones. All of the neurones, or nerve cells are present (millions of them) at birth, however, this does not mean that the new-born's brain is able to function fully.

What is largely missing is the complex system of nerve fibres which transmit messages to and from the brain and between the brain cells. Messages travel from one cell to another via axons, which are fibres going out from the cells, and dendrites, which are extensions of the cells themselves. The all-important junctions between axons and cells are called synapses.

The complexity and efficiency of the brain is a question not simply of the number of cells, but the number of connections that are available to enable message transmission. There is a rapid proliferation in the developing system of nerve fibres during the first two years of life. Another critical feature of brain development is the formation of protective sheaths, of a fatty material called myelin, around the nerve cells. The insulation provided by the myelin sheaths allow messages to be transmitted more rapidly and with greater efficiency.

Myelination is incomplete at birth and develops in different parts of the brain at different times. It is almost complete by the time a child is two, but continues to develop into adolescence. As much of the nerve tissue has little myelin insulation at birth, the rate of nerve transmission is slower in babies than adults and movements are less efficient.

The control of movement improves as myelination of nerves increases and the infant interacts with the environment. The first phase of movement development is the head-to-toe development (cephalocaudal) as a baby shows the ability to control the head and face before the lower limbs. Development is also proximodistal where the development of the midline occurs before the extremities; a baby controls the arm before finer control and manipulation with the fingers.

The development of the brain progresses according to a co-ordinated sequence.

At birth, the cortex—the grey matter that forms the outer surface of the brain and regulates all complex thinking—is barely able to function. Only the parts of the brain that lie below the cortex are effective, and they cannot do much more than command the use of reflexes. As the connections of the cortex form and myelination progresses, the baby's brain becomes more capable of increasing complex operations.

The most active parts of the brain at birth are the sensory-motor cortex, the thalamus, the brain stem and the cerebellum. All the major surface features of the cerebral hemispheres are present at birth, but the cerebral cortex is only half its adult thickness.

The most active parts of baby's brain at birth ▼

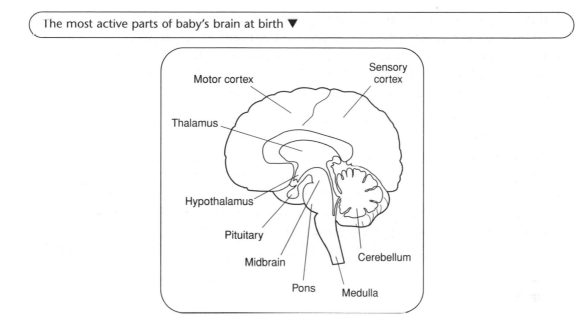

The spinal cord is about 15–18cm long, with its lower end opposite either the second or third lumbar vertebra.

The spinal cord does not grow as much as the vertebral canal and therefore appears to rise as a child grows in length. All the major tracts of the spinal cord are fairly well myelinated, but the motor tracts are less so. However, the local reflexes related to swallowing and sucking appear before birth and have their nerve pathways well myelinated.

Motor development in a baby reflects the neuromuscular maturation and is related to the rapid growth of the brain at this time. The cerebellum controls the development and maintenance of neuromuscular co-ordination, balance and muscle tone. However, the cerebellum starts its growth spurt later than the cerebrum and brain stem but completes it earlier.

The cerebrum and brain stem begin their growth spurt during mid-pregnancy, whereas the cerebellum starts a month or so before full term. By 18 months, the estimated cell count of the cerebellum will have reached adult levels, whereas the cerebellum and brain stem would have only achieved around 60 per cent.

It is during this important development of the cerebellum that the infant develops the postural control and balance required for walking and co-ordinated movements.

Although the brain is programmed to develop in a certain sequence, however the way in which the brain develops is also greatly influenced by how it is nourished, stimulated and protected.

The brain is responsible for the way in which the body works, as it enables babies and children to make sense of the world around them and to store information for future reference. This is why once a skill has been learnt it is important to give babies and children the incentive and opportunity to practise it.

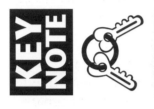

KEY NOTE

> Baby massage is thought to enhance a baby's neurological development and through stimulation of the skin speeds up the myelination of the brain and the nervous system, therefore improving the brain–body communication system.

Reflexes

Reflexes are involuntary responses to stimulation.

New-born babies are equipped with a wide number of primitive reflexes at birth which assist them to survive. Paediatricians use reflexes to help build up a picture of a baby's development.

Some of the reflexes are simple and are mediated at spinal cord level; others are more complex and require the integration of other parts of the brain and developing nervous centres. For instance, primitive reflexes associated with feeding are the rooting, sucking and tongue retrusion reflex which are well developed at birth and are permanent.

The Startle or 'Moro' reflex, where a startled baby will throw out his legs and arms and arch his back in response to a sudden change in his position or a loud noise, lasts until around 3–4 months of age.

A second set of reflexes, the locomotor reflexes, resemble later voluntary movements and allow a child to move through space. These include creeping, standing, stepping and swimming. These movements do not include voluntary control at first but during infancy they gradually diminish and are integrated into voluntary patterns.

A third group of reflexes in the new-born are the postural reflexes. An example of this is the tonic neck reflex. This develops in the first few months of life. When a baby's head is turned to one side he or she responds with an increased muscle tone and extension of both the arm and leg of the opposite side.

The Cardiovascular System in Babies

Circulation changes occur in the heart at birth as babies start to depend on their lungs for oxygen, rather than their mother's placenta.

The Fetal Circulation

The fetal circulation differs from that of an adult in that the lungs, digestive organs and kidneys are non-functional, and only begin functioning at birth. The foetus therefore receives its oxygen and nutrients by diffusion from the maternal circulation, with metabolic waste products being removed by the maternal circulation.

The foetus is connected to the mother's uterus by a long **umbilical cord** that terminates in the **placenta**. The placenta and the umbilical cord provide the two-way route by which oxygen, nutrients and other materials pass from the mother to the foetus and waste and cellular secretions pass from the foetus to the maternal circulation.

The fetal circulation is therefore modified to reflect the non-functional respiratory system and the connection with the placenta.

Blood passes from the foetus to the placenta via two **umbilical arteries**, which are branches of the **internal iliac arteries** (branches of the aorta). At the placenta waste products are deposited, and oxygen and nutrients are obtained.

The umbilical arteries wind together through the umbilical cord. At the placenta, they divide into many branches that form smaller vessels where exchange takes place.

After the exchanges have occurred, the blood rich in oxygen and nutrients emerges from the placenta and is returned to the foetus through a single large **umbilical vein**, which extends through the umbilical cord. As the umbilical vein enters the foetus it ascends to the level of the liver. The umbilical vein branches upon contact with the fetal liver and most of the blood flows into a vein called the **ductus venosus**, which passes through the liver and joins the fetal inferior vena cava. Placental blood entering the inferior vena cava joins blood from other tissues and pours into the right atrium of the fetal heart.

Blood entering the fetal right atrium from the superior vena cava is low in oxygen and laden with waste products, while blood from the inferior vena cava is rich in oxygen and nutrients from the placenta. Blood from these two sources mixes in the right atrium.

Some of the blood, primarily that from the superior vena cava, flows through the tricuspid valve into the right ventricle. However some of the blood, primarily from the inferior vena cava passes, through an opening between the atria called the **foramen ovale** that diverts blood directly into the left atrium, bypassing the right ventricle. This blood flows into the left ventricle, bypassing the pulmonary circulation and hence the lungs.

Blood in the right ventricle is pumped into the pulmonary trunk when the heart contracts. Instead of going to the lungs, however, most of it is diverted to the aorta through a short valve called the **ductus arteriosus**, which shunts blood directly into the aorta at the superior surface of the heart. The ductus arteriosus prevents blood from going into the lungs and sends it directly to the aorta for distribution to the body. The blood in the aorta is carried to all parts of the foetus through the systemic circulation.

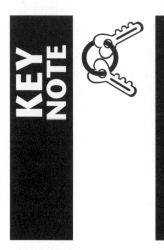

KEY NOTE

In an adult, venous blood entering the right atrium flows to the right ventricle into the pulmonary trunk. In the fetal heart, much of the blood in the right ventricle is diverted away from the largely non-functional pulmonary circuit as the fetal respiratory system is not active.

The net effect of the modifications in the fetal circulation is to divert blood away from the non-functioning pulmonary system into the systemic circulation. Functionally, this increases the amount of blood sent through the placenta, thereby increasing the efficiency in the exchange of materials between the foetus and its mother.

Circulation Changes That Occur in Babies After Birth

Immediately after birth, the following changes occur:

✳ Blood begins flowing through the pulmonary circulation when the ductus arteriosus contracts by vasoconstriction, atrophies and becomes the ligamentum arteriosum.

✳ In addition to this, the foramen ovale closes to become the fossa ovalis, a depression in the interatria septum.

✳ The right and left atria become completely separated from one another.

✳ The umbilical vessels undergo degeneration and the digestive and renal arteries and veins begin functioning.

At birth, when an infant takes its first breath, the alveoli in the lungs fill with air and the constricted pulmonary vessels open to allow more blood to flow into the lungs. At the same time the umbilical flow is stopped.

The pressure changes and the reduction of the prostraglandins that maintained the pregnancy causes the ductus arteriosus and foramen ovale to close.

The mass of the heart in babies in relation to body mass is high, but reduces as childhood progresses.

Infants have smaller hearts that have to beat faster to oxygenate their body tissues.

A pulse rate of a new-born is around 145; at 6 months this decrease to 120, and at one year 115.

The Respiratory System in Babies

The lungs of a foetus are filled with fluid until delivery, and as the baby is squeezed through the vaginal canal the lungs are gradually squeezed of fluid.

Any residual fluid is absorbed through the pulmonary capillaries and into the lymphatics.

The combination of reduced oxygen levels, acidity and rising carbon dioxide levels in the blood, along with light, sound and touch activate the central and peripheral arterial chemoreceptors, which stimulate a baby to take its first breath.

As the lungs expand the pulmonary arterioles dilate and blood flows into the lungs. The lungs then recoil away from the chest wall due to the elastic fibres in the lung tissue, and the chest wall will spring out.

There follows a transition of breathing from irregular, ineffectual movements at birth to regular, rhythmic effort by the end of a baby's first week.

Babies breathe though their noses up to four weeks of age. They have small airways that narrow further when swollen or blocked with mucus secretions.

Babies therefore do not adapt well to mouth breathing and airway resistance in children is high due to the small diameter of their respiratory tree.

The respiratory tract is very short in a baby and therefore the risk of infective material entering it is high. Also, due to the respiratory structures being small and situated close together, respiratory infections causing inflammation of the mucosa of the nasal passages and pharynx will soon involve other associated structures such as the ear.

The tonsils and adenoids are areas of lymphatic tissue that are the first line of defence in the respiratory system. They are situated in the throat and at the back of the nose and have an important function in helping protect children from infection.

They can become enlarged and cause discomfort.

Areolar tissue exists in the vocal cords of young children (which is not present in an adult) and will subsequently swell and block the trachea if inflamed. Children and babies have short slender vocal cords and therefore their voices tend to be high pitched.

A baby's trachea is very elastic and flexible, and is situated high at the third thoracic vertebral level. There is therefore a great need to support their heads and position them with the jaw at right angles to the spine.

Small children also lose more water and body heat from the body tissues in breathing and are more likely to develop mucus plugs along with respiratory infections.

Small babies are highly susceptible to viruses and bacteria (droplet spread infections) e.g. colds and meningitis.

In a small baby the respiratory system is less efficient than in an adult as the diaphragm is more horizontal and the lower ribs are retracted when lying supine. This means the diaphragm will need greater effort to generate tidal volume.

In babies the glottis is positioned towards the head, the laryngeal reflexes are more active and the epiglottis is longer. This is very significant in the positioning of resuscitation for a child.

After birth, the airways increase in length and diameter and continue to mature until about the age of eight, when the respiratory tree is complete.

The Digestive System in Babies

After a baby is born it is suddenly separated from its source of nutrients in the maternal circulation. It is therefore not uncommon for the newborn baby to lose 5–10 per cent of its body weight due to shock of birth. At birth an infant's lips are well adapted to closing round a nipple or bottle to feed.

Prior to birth the gastrointestinal tract is filled with fluid and the remnants of the developing bowel lumen as it grows and sheds the lining. During the first few breaths after birth the infant swallows air and within a few hours the whole gut contains gas. Therefore as the infant feeds, a large volume of gas is taken in, causing wind.

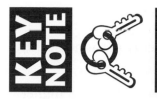

KEY NOTE

The best position to wind a baby after a feed is to hold them sitting and supported at the back and neck to allow the gas to bubble up a straight oesophagus.

The stomach is positioned high in the abdomen in infants and is placed transversely, rather than vertically as in older children. The capacity of the stomach changes with age. A new-born may only take 10–20ml; a 1-month baby 90–150ml and a baby of one year 210–360ml! A new-born stomach is emptied every two-and-a-half to three hours.

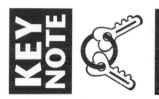

KEY NOTE

It is important for parents to note that as a new-born's stomach is emptied so frequently, there is little point feeding every hour as this may encourage posseting.

At birth the abdomen and thorax are of equal circumference. As the muscles in the body are all poorly developed the abdomen will appear prominent.

At birth approximately 40 per cent of the peritoneal cavity is occupied by the liver, which displaces the bowel. The hepatic flexure of the colon moves to lie at a lower level than the splenic flexure. The transverse colon moves higher and the small bowel lies centrally in the abdomen.

The liver is functionally immature in a new-born, as it lacks sufficient enzymes required for the production of bilirubin. The enzyme system usually develops within two weeks of birth. This explains why jaundice is a common problem in the first two weeks of a baby's life.

Small babies cannot control their bowel movements until their central nervous system has matured enough to allow them better control. A stool is therefore passed in response to the rectum being full.

The stool of a new-born is known as meconium. They are dark-green, odourless and have a smooth, paste-like appearance. They are composed of digestive juices, desquamated cells and amniotic fluid which is passed in the baby's first few days of life.

Stools after this are yellow in colour and are slightly porridge-like with a sour smell and may be passed several times a day if the baby is breast fed. Faeces consist of water, casein, fat, fatty acids, mineral salts, live and dead bacteria.

The Renal System in Babies

The renal system is of major importance in childhood as it is critical to the healthy functioning of all body systems.

Water makes up about 70 per cent of an infant's body tissues and there is a higher turnover of water due to increased heat production and an immature kidney function to conserve water.

Infants and young children have a larger blood volume circulating per kilogram of body weight. However, their overall body volume is small, so loss of blood volume will naturally have a more devastating effect and affect vital organs more quickly.

Infants take water in from their diet and this controlled automatically by thirst, a dry mouth and the stimulation of the hypothalamus.

Infants also produce water as a by-product of their higher metabolic rate. They lose water mainly through their large skin surface, more rapid breathing and relatively longer intestines.

The kidney of a new-born baby weighs around 23g, which will double in size by 6 months and treble by the end of the first year of life. The new-born's kidney has millions of tiny filtration units (nephrons) which although immature at birth gradually increase their capacity for filtration.

In the infant the bladder sits higher in the abdominal cavity and descends into the pelvis as more space becomes available. The posterior surface of the bladder is completely covered by the peritoneum. The bladder is shaped like a cigar and does not achieve its adult pyramid shape until about six years of age.

The ureter in an infant is relatively shorter than that in an older child and has no pelvic portion. A baby is incapable of exercising any control over their bladder. The bladder will voluntarily empty when stretched by a volume of 15ml (the adult volume is 200ml). When the bladder fills it distends and sends impulses to the sacral area of the spine via the autonomic nervous system. Motor impulses from the spinal cord via the autonomic nervous system initiate relaxation of the internal sphincter and contraction of detensor muscle (muscle of the urinary bladder wall) leading to urine being expelled.

Bladder control requires the necessary nervous systems' development in order that sensory impulses can travel via the spinal cord to the central micturition control centre in the brain. Successful control of the bladder usually starts at about two years of age when the child can voluntarily relax the pelvic floor muscles.

The Reproductive System in Babies

In the first few weeks of gestation, the foetus has an 'indifferent' gonad, which comprises of two layers, an outer cortex and an inner medulla. If male, the medulla forms a testis to determine the male sexual organs, while the cortex disappears under the influence of the testis-determining factor on the Y chromosome to determine the genetic sex. If no Y chromosome is present, the cortex will develop and the embryo will continue to develop as a female.

The anatomy of the reproductive tract develops in the male and female at different times. At 8 to 12 weeks testosterone will have stimulated growth of the male reproductive system, and the epididymis, vas deferens. Bulbourethral glands and the seminal vesicle will be complete by 15 weeks. By the third month of gestation the female system is developed. The fallopian tubes, uterus and inner section of the vagina are complete.

In the male, the cells that produce sperm remain dormant from the seventh week of embryonic development until puberty. In the female, under influence of the two X chromosomes, the primordial germ cells undergo a few more mitotic divisions after this time to develop eggs. They commence meiotic division by the fifth month of fetal life. They then also remain dormant until puberty.

Changes that Occur in the Reproductive System at Birth

In the male, the testicles usually descend through the inguinal canal to the scrotum, as the abdominal viscera and testosterone action increases.

The descent of the testicles is a necessary stage for the maturation of the sperm at a later stage (which require a cooler temperature than body heat). The seminiferous tubules are solid at birth and will not enlarge and canalise until the testicles enlarge at puberty. The weight of an adult testicle is around 40 times that of a new-born baby.

The prostate gland and the rectum are the two major organs that occupy the pelvis at birth. The prostate grows slowly until puberty and then doubles in size over a short period of time. The penis is relatively large in the new-born baby, with the foreskin separated from the glans.

In the female the ovaries are small at birth, but are large in comparison to the testicles. They consist of around 400,000 eggs at birth which then decline in number over childhood. They lie in the abdominal cavity in the infant and only enter the ovarian fossae at approximately six years of age as the bladder descends into the pelvis. The ovarian tissue will grow to 20 times its weight up until; puberty, when the remaining egg release is stimulated by the hypothalamus.

The uterus appears large at birth due to the influence of the maternal hormones through the placenta and the cervix size is larger than the uterus. The uterus lies in the same plane as the vagina until the bladder descends at around six years of age.

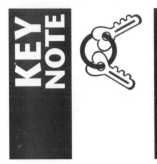

KEY NOTE

Enlarged genitals and breasts are common in both sexes in the period immediately after birth. The breasts may even ooze a little milk, and baby girls may have a slight vaginal discharge.

This is caused by maternal hormones circulating the blood stream and the effects will disappear in the first few weeks of the baby's life.

The Immune System in Babies

The immune response is activated by specialised types of white blood bells called lymphocytes. There are two types of lymphocytes: B-cells which produce chemicals called antibodies, and T-cells which interact directly with the invading antigen (any substance the body regards as foreign or potentially dangerous).

The lymphocytes are found in the blood, bone marrow, the thymus, the lymph nodes, the spleen and the tissue spaces. The thymus gland (a bilobed organ found in the root of the neck, above and in front of the heart) is significant in infancy, in that it controls the development of lymphoid tissue and the immune response to microbes and foreign proteins. T-Lymphocytes migrate from the bone marrow to the thymus, where they mature and differentiate until they are activated by antigen.

The thymus gland produces thymic hormones which help infants and children make antibodies. In relation to body size, the thymus is largest at birth. It remains large throughout infancy and childhood and shrinks in adult life.

The immune system starts developing early in intra-uterine life, and by the fifteenth week about 65 per cent of the lymphocytes in the fetal thymus are T-cells.

Lymph vessels develop in the fifth and sixth week of embryonic development and start joining together to form a closed network of lymphatics and lymph sacs. A baby's lymph glands are present at birth. However, despite this, babies still have immature immune responses, as their immune systems take many years to develop. This makes them a very susceptible target host group to a range of childhood infections and illnesses.

Babies are born with *passive* immunity, as immunoglobulins (antibodies) pass from the mother to the foetus across the placenta. B-cells secrete a number of antibodies, or immunoglobulins. IgG is the major immunoglobulin found in lymphoid tissue and represents 75 per cent of all immunoglobulins. It passes from blood to interstitial spaces, and moves through the placenta to provide the foetus and new-born with maternally acquired immunity for the first three months of life, while the baby's own production rises. It is present in high concentrations in colostrum (the first secretion from the breast, occurring shortly after, or sometimes before birth, prior to the secretion of true milk) and breast milk. Therefore, this type of acquired immunity is short lived.

KEY NOTE

During pregnancy a blood test is taken to check a mother's blood group and whether the blood is rhesus negative or positive. A few mothers may be rhesus negative; this is significant as when the mother is pregnant with an Rh positive foetus, small amounts of Rh-positive blood from the foetus may leak into the maternal circulation. If the mother is exposed to the Rh-positive cells, she develops antibodies against the Rh antigen. Usually the first foetus is not harmed by the antigen-antibody reaction as the leakage tends to occur at the time of delivery and not many antibodies are developed by the mother. If the mother becomes pregnant again with an Rh-positive foetus, the antibodies that she has already developed can enter the fetal circulation and causes agglutination (clumping) and haemolysis (destruction) of the fetal blood cells. This is known as haemolytic disease of the new-born and if the reaction is severe, the foetus can die in the uterus, or if less severe, develop anaemia or jaundice. Fortunately, injecting anti-Rh antibodies into the Rh-negative mother soon after delivery can prevent the development of antibodies. These anti-Rh antibodies recognise Rh antigens, and if they enter, they destroy them before they can stimulate the immune system in the mother.

Active immunity arises when the body's own cells produce and remain able to produce appropriate antibodies following exposure to an infection such as the common cold or chickenpox, or by artificial immunisation or vaccination against measles, mumps and rubella (MMR).

Immunisation stimulates the immune system in the following ways. Live weakened pathogenic micro-organisms stimulate the body to recognise a foreign antigen and produce antibodies to destroy it. The memory created protects a child from future invasion of the particular pathogen. An example of this is the MMR vaccination, which can induce a mild form of measles within ten days of the immunisation or create a general inflammatory response.

Modified bacterial toxins (such as those from tetanus and diptheria) are made non-toxic and retain the ability to stimulate the formation of antibodies

Dead organisms are injected, which have the 'shape' of the antigen, but cannot divide and multiply in the body. The lymphocytes then recognise them as foreign, producing a memory cell for future attacks. Vaccinations for typhoid and whooping cough (pertussis) are used in this way.

Immunisation Programme for Infants ▼	
At 2 months	Diphtheria Whooping Cough Tetanus Hib Polio Meningitis C
At 3 months	Diphtheria Whooping Cough Tetanus Hib Polio Meningitis C
At 4 months	Diphtheria Whooping Cough Tetanus Hib Polio Meningitis C
At 12–15 months	Measles Mumps Rubella (MMR)
At 3–5 years (pre-school booster)	Diphtheria Tetanus Polio

Diphtheria: an acute highly contagious bacterial infection, which starts with a sore throat and then quickly develops into a serious illness which blocks the nose and throat, making it difficult and sometimes nearly impossible for the child to breathe.

Fortunately an effective immunisation programme has made diphtheria rare in most western countries.

Tetanus: an acute infectious disease, which occurs by contamination of wounds by bacterial spores. It attacks the nervous system causing painful muscle spasms.

Immunisation has made tetanus rare, but there is still a chance of contracting it.

Whooping Cough: a highly contagious bacterial infection, which affects the respiratory tract. It causes long bouts of severe coughing and choking, leaving the sufferer exhausted. Whooping cough can cause convulsions, ear infections, pneumonia, bronchitis, and even brain damage.

Immunisation offers effective protection and is usually given in the form of the DPT vaccine.

Haemophilus influenzae type b (Hib): the commonest form of bacterial meningitis in the under-fives. It causes epiglottitis (a severe form of croup), pneumonia, blood poisoning, and infections of the bones and joints. It affects babies under a year more severely and can be fatal.

Before the introduction of the Hib vaccine in the UK in 1992, Hib was the commonest cause of meningitis in children under the age of two.

Polio: a viral infection of the central nervous system, which causes muscle paralysis. Fortunately polio is extremely rare in western countries, due to an effective immunisation programme. The disease is most common where sanitation is poor as the virus is excreted in the faeces of an infected person. There is, therefore, still risk of contact with the disease through foreign travel.

Measles: a highly infectious viral disease. It begins like a bad cold with a fever and then a rash appears which is often accompanied by a bad cough and high temperature. If severe, measles can cause convulsions, ear infections, bronchitis and pneumonia. Vaccination against measles provides effective immunity.

Meningitis: an acute inflammation of the membranes that cover the brain and spinal cord, which requires immediate medical treatment. Meningitis most frequently results from an infection, either bacterial or viral.

Viral meningitis occurs most commonly after mumps, but is not as serious as bacterial meningitis.

Bacterial meningitis is serious, but can be treated with antibiotics if it is diagnosed early enough. The symptoms of meningitis are a fever, stiff neck, lethargy, headaches, drowsiness and intolerance to bright lights. In some cases there may be a purple-red rash.

Children are now offered Hib vaccinations against two types of meningitis.

Mumps: a common virus infection commonly affecting school-age children. Symptoms appear two to three weeks after exposure and may include a fever, headache, and vomiting, in addition to the typical swelling of the parotid salivary glands. The parotid glands on the side of the face often swell up.

Vaccination against mumps provides effective immunity.

Rubella (German Measles): a mild highly contagious virus infection causing enlargement of the lymph nodes in the neck and a widespread pink rash. Although usually a mild disease, it is one which can harm an unborn baby if a woman catches it whilst pregnant. The risk is particularly high during the first four months of pregnancy. Babies whose mothers contract rubella during pregnancy can be born deaf, blind, and with heart and brain damage.

Most children receive effective immunisation via the MMR vaccine in their second year.

Questions for Review

1. State two factors that affect a baby's skeletal development

   _____

   _____

2. State the reason why babies' heads look out of proportion to their bodies in the first year of life

   _____

   _____

3. The changes in posture of a baby during its first year of life are due to the development of the ……………….   ………………….. in the spine

4. State why it is important to take care to avoid applying too much pressure when massaging young babies

   _____

   _____

   _____

   _____

5. What are the fontanelles and what is their significance in baby massage?

   _____

   _____

   _____

   _____

6. State which parts of a baby's skeleton are made of cartilage and do not turn into bone until adolescence

   _____

   _____

   _____

   _____

7. At what age do a baby's skull bones fuse together?

_____

_____

8. Why do babies/small children have a lot of infections/runny noses?

_____

_____

_____

9. At what age do a baby's primary teeth generally start to erupt?

_____

_____

_____

10. Put the following types of teeth in the order in which they develop in babies: four lateral incisors, back molars, four front molars, upper central incisors, canines, lower central incisors

_____

_____

_____

_____

11. i) Describe a baby's muscle fibres at birth.

    ii) How does this affect the application of massage movements?

_____

_____

_____

_____

_____

_____

_____

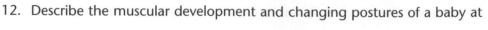

12. Describe the muscular development and changing postures of a baby at

   i) 3 months

   _____

   _____

   ii) 6 months

   _____

   _____

   iii) 8–9 months

   _____

   _____

   iv) one year

   _____

   _____

13. State the three most important factors affecting muscle development in babies

   _____

   _____

14. Describe how massage can help a baby's muscular development

   _____

   _____

   _____

   _____

15. Which muscles take until approximately 18 months to two years to become under the conscious control of a baby?

   _____

   _____

16. i) Why is a new-born baby's skin extremely sensitive to touch?

_____

_____

ii) Explain how the above factor influences massage of young babies

_____

_____

17. A baby's tissues are initially made up of a high proportion of ....

18. Explain why babies need to be kept warm

_____

_____

_____

_____

19. i) What does a baby's nervous tissue lack at birth?

_____

_____

ii) How does this influence a baby's movements?

_____

_____

20. List the most active parts of a baby's brain at birth

_____

_____

21. Which part of the brain is responsible for postural control and balance in babies?

_____

_____

22. State two ways in which brain development may be influenced in babies

_____

_____

23. Explain how baby massage is thought to enhance a baby's neurological development

_____

_____

_____

_____

_____

_____

24. How does fetal circulation differ from an adult's circulatory system?

_____

_____

_____

_____

_____

_____

25. State the circulation changes that occur in babies following birth

_____

_____

_____

_____

_____

_____

_____

_____

_____

26. Why do baby's hearts beat faster?

_____

_____

_____

_____

27. Why is the risk of infective material entering a baby's respiratory system high?

_____

_____

_____

_____

28. State two differences in a baby's respiratory system compared to an adult's

_____

_____

_____

_____

29. Why do babies' and small children's voices tend to be high pitched?

_____

_____

_____

_____

30. Why is a small baby's respiratory system less efficient than an adult's?

_____

_____

_____

_____

31. At what age does a child's respiratory system mature?

_____

_____

32. How does the position of the stomach differ in infants, as compared to older children and adults?

_____

_____

_____

_____

33. Why does the abdomen appear prominent in babies?

_____

_____

34. Why is jaundice a common problem in the first two weeks of a baby's life?

_____

_____

35. Why are small babies unable to control their bowel movements?

_____

_____

36. Why is the renal system of major importance in childhood?

_____

_____

37. State two reasons why infants have a high turnover of water in their bodies.

_____

_____

_____

_____

38. How does the position *and* shape of the bladder in babies differ from adults?

_____

_____

_____

_____

39. State the changes that occur in the reproductive system in babies at birth

    i) changes in the male

_____

_____

_____

_____

_____

_____

    ii) changes in the female

_____

_____

_____

_____

_____

_____

40. Why are enlarged genitals and breasts common in both sexes following birth and during the first few weeks of life?

_____

_____

_____

_____

41. i) Which gland is significant in immunity during infancy?

_____

_____

_____

ii) What is its function?

_____

_____

_____

_____

42. Briefly explain how babies are provided with

i) passive immunity

_____

_____

_____

_____

ii) active immunity

_____

_____

_____

_____

Baby Growth and Development 05

Baby Growth and Development

Growth and development is remarkably rapid during the first two years of a baby's life. This chapter explores the fascinating aspects of physical, social and emotional development of babies from birth to 18 months. Although the development sections are dealt with separately in this chapter, it is important for both instructors and parents to consider all aspects of child development as a whole.

A baby's development will also be largely influenced by genetic inheritance, as well as social and environmental influences. Having an understanding of child development in the early years will help instructors and parents to recognise the changing postures of the infant and how this influences massage positioning, and how social interaction is enhanced through the massage session.

By the end of this chapter you will be able to relate the following knowledge in your role as instructor/parent/carer.

* The physical development of babies
* The social and emotional development of babies
* Bonding and attachment
* Language development in babies
* Cognitive development in babies

Physical Development

Physical development refers to the way in which the body increases in skills and becomes more complex in its performance.

The progress of muscular movement is called motor development and may be divided into:

* gross motor skills that involve whole body movements (sitting, crawling, walking)

✱ fine motor skills which involve hand-eye co-ordination (holding and exploring objects).

At Birth (New-born)

Gross Motor Development

Typical postures of new-born babies include the following.

Prone (baby lying face down)

✱ Baby lies with head to one side, resting on the cheek

✱ Body assumes a frog-like posture with the bottom up and the knees curled up under the tummy

✱ The arms are bent at the elbows and tucked under the chest with the fists clenched

Posture of a new-born (baby lying face down) ▼

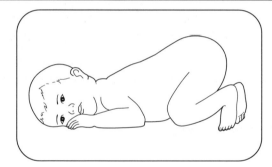

Supine (baby lying on the back)

✱ Baby lies with the head to one side

✱ Knees are bent towards the body, with the soles of the feet touching

✱ Arms are bent inwards towards the body

✱ Baby's movements are jerky and random (kicking with the feet)

Posture of a new-born (baby lying face up) ▼

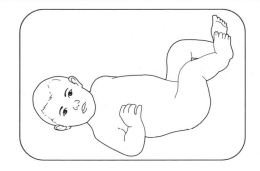

Ventral suspension (held in the air face down)

❋ Baby's head and legs fall below the level of the back, so that the baby makes a complete downwards curve

Sitting

❋ When the baby is pulled upwards to a sitting position, there is complete head lag. Baby's head falls backwards as the body comes up and then flops forward onto the chest

❋ If the baby is held in a sitting position, the back is completely curved and the head is on the chest

Fine Motor Development

❋ Baby's fists are clenched

❋ Baby concentrates on carer's face when feeding

❋ Baby can focus on 15–25cm range and will stare at brightly coloured mobiles within visual range

1-Month-Old Baby

Typical postures of 1-month-old babies include the following:

Gross motor development

Prone (lying face down)

❋ Baby lies with head to one side but can now lift head to change position

❋ Legs are bent and no longer tucked under the body

❋ Arms are bent away from the body, with the hands usually closed

Supine (lying on the back)

* Baby's head is on one side
* The arm and leg on the side the head is facing will stretch out
* Both arms may be bent, with legs bent at knees, soles of the feet facing each other

Ventral suspension (held in the air face down)

* The head is on the same level as the back and the legs are coming up towards the level of the back

Sitting

* If the baby is pulled to sit, the head will lag and fall backwards. However, it will remain steady for a moment as sitting position is achieved, but will fall forwards
* Back is a complete curve when held in a sitting position

Posture of a 1-month-old baby (sitting) ▼

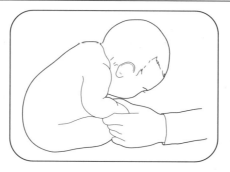

Fine Motor Development

At 1 month a baby will:

* Turn its head towards the light and stare at bright shiny objects
* Follow bright moving objects within 5-10cm from the face
* Gaze attentively at their carer's face whilst being fed
* Grasp a finger or other object placed in the hand
* Hands will usually be closed

Baby at 3 Months

Gross Motor Development

Typical postures of a 3-month-old baby include the following.

Prone (lying face down)

* Baby can now lift up the head and chest supported on the elbows, forearms and hands

* Bottom assumes a flatter position, with the legs straighter and kicking alternately

* Baby may scratch at the floor and bob the head in a rocking motion

Posture of a 3-month-old baby (lying face down) ▼

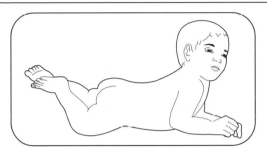

Supine (lying on the back)

* Baby usually lies with the head in a central position

* The movements of the legs and arms are now more smooth and continuous

* The legs can kick strongly; sometimes together and sometimes alternately

* The baby brings their hands together over the body and waves the arms asymmetrically

Posture of a 3-month-baby (lying face up) ▼

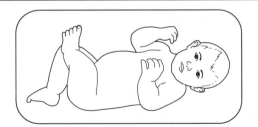

Ventral suspension (held in the air face down)

* The head is now held above the level of the back and the legs are on the same level

Sitting

* When the baby is pulled to sit, the head should come forwards steadily with the back

* The head may fall forwards after a short time in the sitting position
* There should be little or no head lag at three months
* When held in a sitting position the back should be straight, except for a curve in the lumbar region

> Posture of a 3-month-old baby (sitting) ▼

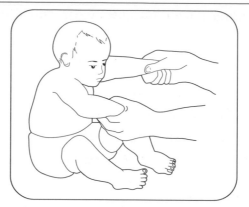

Standing

* When held in a standing position the baby will sag at the knees
* The placing and walking reflexes should have disappeared

Fine Motor Development

At 3 months a baby typically:

* Plays with their fingers
* Holds a rattle or similar object for a short time when placed in the hand
* Recognises the bottle or breast and waves the arms around in excitement

6-Month-Old Baby

Gross Motor Development

Typical postures of a 6-month-old baby include the following:

Prone (lying face down)

* The baby can now lift the head and chest wall clear of the floor by supporting themselves on outstretched arms (hands are flat on the floor)
* Can roll over from front to back
* May pull the knees up in an attempt to crawl, but will slide backwards

Supine (lying on the back)

✳ The baby will lift the head to look at the feet

✳ May lift the arms, requesting to be picked up

✳ Will kick the legs strongly

✳ May roll over from back to front

✳ May lift up the legs, grasp one or both of the legs and attempt to put them in the mouth

Sitting

✳ When pulled to sit, the baby can grab an adult's hands and pull themselves into a sitting position (head is now fully controlled by strong neck muscles)

✳ Can sit with the back straight for long periods with support

✳ May sit for short periods without support, but will topple over easily

Posture of a 6-month-old baby (sitting) ▼

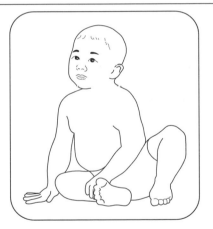

Standing

✳ If held standing, the baby will enjoy bouncing up and down

✳ When held in the air and whooshed down feet first, may demonstrate the parachute reflex when the legs will straighten and separate and the toes fan out

Fine Motor Development

At 6 months a baby typically:

✳ Transfers a toy or object from hand to hand

✳ Puts items in the mouth in order to explore them

❋ Is fascinated by small toys within reaching distance and will grab them using the palmar grasp (whole hand grasp)

❋ Appears bright and alert looking around to take in all the visual information in the environment

❋ Watches an item or toy falling when dropped, if it is within sight (if it falls out of a sight a baby of this age will not look for it)

9-Month-Old Baby

Gross Motor Development

Typical postures of a 9-month-old baby include the following:

Prone (lying face down)

❋ The baby may be able to support the body on knees and outstretched arms

❋ May rock backwards and forwards and try to crawl

❋ Move backwards in the crawling position

Posture of a 9-month-old baby (crawling) ▼

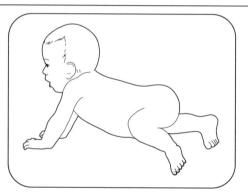

Supine (lying on the back)

❋ Baby may roll from back to front and may crawl away, roll around the floor or squirm around on the back

Sitting

❋ The baby may sit unsupported for 15 minutes or more

❋ Will keep their balance when turning to reach for toys from the side

❋ Will put their arms out to prevent falling

❋ May begin to bottom shuffle, moving around the floor in an upright sitting position

Standing

✳ Baby can pull themselves to a standing position

✳ When supported by an adult, can step forward on alternate feet

✳ Will support the body in a standing position by holding on to a firm object

✳ May begin to side step around furniture

✳ Cannot lower themselves onto the floor and will fall backwards onto the bottom

✳ May begin to crawl upstairs but is unable to get down safely

Fine Motor Development

At 9 months a baby typically:

✳ Uses a pincer grasp with the index finger and thumb

✳ Drops objects or bangs them onto a hard surface to release them (cannot let go of items voluntarily yet)

✳ Looks for fallen objects out of sight

✳ Is visually alert and curious, exploring objects before picking them up

✳ Grasps objects, usually with one hand, inspecting them with the eyes and transferring them to the other hand

✳ May hold one object in each hand and bang them together

✳ Uses the index finger to poke and point

12-Month-Old Baby

Gross Motor Development

Typical postures of a 12-month-old baby include:

Sitting

The baby can typically:

✳ Sit alone indefinitely

✳ Get into a sitting position from lying down

Standing

The baby can:

✳ Pull themselves up to stand and walk around furniture

✳ Return to sitting without falling

✳ (May) stand alone for a short period of time

> Posture of a 12-month baby (standing) ▼

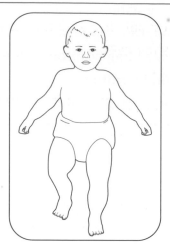

Mobility

✴ At 12 months the baby is now mobile by either crawling, bottom-shuffling, walking alone or with one or both hands held

✴ May crawl upstairs forwards and downstairs backwards

Fine Motor Development

A 12-month-old baby:

✴ Looks for objects hidden and out of sight

✴ Uses a mature pincer grasps and releases objects

✴ Throws toys deliberately and watches them fall

✴ Likes to point at picture books and points at familiar objects

✴ Clasps hands together in delight and in play

Baby at 15-Months-Old

Gross Motor Development

Typical postures of a 15-month-old baby include:

✴ Walks alone, with feet wide apart with arms raised to maintain balance

✴ Falls easily, sometimes after a few paces and usually on stopping

✴ Sits from standing by falling backwards onto the bottom or forwards onto the arms

- Stands without help of furniture or people
- Kneels without support
- May climb forwards onto a small chair and turn to sit
- Throw back a ball (but may fall over)
- Climbs the stairs on all fours

Posture of a 15-month-old baby (walking) ▼

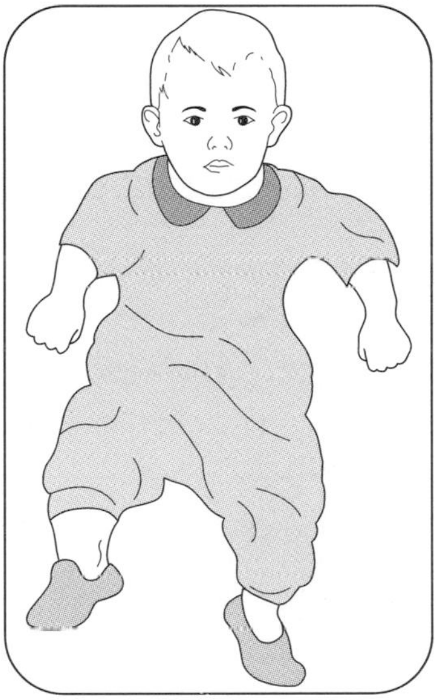

Fine Motor Development

- Enjoys playing with small bricks and building a small tower
- Enjoys brightly coloured books and turns several pages at once
- Points at familiar objects in a book and pats the page
- Holds a spoon and puts it to the mouth (may put it in upside down)
- Uses the index finger to constantly demand drinks, food and toys out of reach
- Holds a crayon in a palmar grasp, scribbling backwards and forwards
- Stares out of the window for long periods watching and pointing at activities with interest

18 Months

Gross Motor Development

Typical postures of an 18-month-old include the following:

* Walks confidently, now without using the arms for balance
* Squats to the floor to pick up toys
* Tries to kick a ball
* Likes pushing a brick trolley or wheeled toy
* Walks upstairs or downstairs with hand held
* Comes downstairs either forwards on the bottom, or backwards crawling, or sliding on the tummy
* Runs, but will often fall as at this age babies are unable to co-ordinate movements to get around objects in the way

Posture of a 18-month-old baby (running) ▼

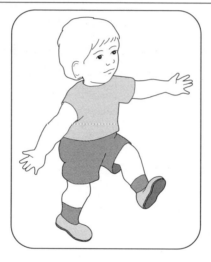

Fine Motor Development

At 18 months a baby:

* Now uses a delicate and refined pincer grasp to put small objects through small spaces
* Scribbles to and fro on paper
* Builds a higher tower block with cubes or bricks
* Tries to thread large beads
* Continues to enjoy picture books and point at known objects

Social and Emotional Development

Social development relates to the growth of a child's ability to relate to others appropriately, and become independent within a social framework. It encompasses:

✻ The growth of a child's relationships with others

✻ The development of social skills and socialisation that lead to independence.

Emotional development is the growth of a child's ability to feel and express an increasing range of emotions in an appropriate way. It encompasses:

✻ The development of feeling towards other people

✻ The growth of a child's feelings and an awareness of themselves

✻ The development of self-image and self-identity.

It is important to remember when studying different types of development (physical, social, emotional and language) that it is a whole process, as all areas of a child's development are integrated and will be affected by each other.

Social and Emotional Development at Birth

New-born babies begin to learn as soon as they are born, however at this stage their behaviour and communication is limited. In general, new-born babies will cry in order to make their needs known and are generally peaceful when their needs are met.

At this stage babies

✻ are completely dependent on others

✻ have rooting, sucking and swallowing reflexes

✻ sleep most of the time

✻ prefer to be left undisturbed

✻ startle at noise, and turn to the light, providing it is not too bright

✻ are usually in close contact with their carer.

Social and Emotional Development at 1 Month

✻ At one month, babies learn to smile at a voice and a face and are attracted to the movement of faces

✻ Around this age babies

  ✻ sleep for most of the time when not being fed or handled

  ✻ cry for their needs to be attended to (different cries are evident for hunger, pain, discomfort, boredom etc)

  ✻ will turn to the breast

  ✻ will look briefly at a human face

  ✻ will quieten in response to their main carer's voice

✽ will smile in response to main care's voice

✽ develop a social smile and respond with vocalisations to the sight and sound of a person (around 6 weeks)

✽ grasp a finger if the hand is opened and the palm is touched.

Social and Emotional Development at 2 Months

✽ At 2 months babies begin to learn a range of responses and behaviour as a result of physical maturation and beginning to explore their environment.

✽ At 2 months a baby is capable of having 'conversations' with the carer; these are a mixture of gestures and noises, but will follow the pattern in that one person is quiet while the other speaks.

✽ Around this stage babies:

  ✽ stop crying when they are picked up

  ✽ sleep less during the day and more at night

  ✽ follow a human face when it moves

  ✽ smile and become responsive to others

  ✽ explore using the five senses

  ✽ differentiate between objects, and begin to tell one face from another.

Social and Emotional Development at 3 Months

✽ At 3 months babies take a lot of interest in their environment and begin to rapidly learn a range of social skills from the people around them. They turn their heads in response to different sounds and to see what people are doing.

✽ Even at this early stage it is essential that someone takes time to communicate with the baby. Babies appear to have a natural capacity to communicate, however this cannot develop without contact and interaction from others.

✽ Around this age babies:

  ✽ respond to friendly handling and smile at most people

  ✽ use sounds to interact socially and reach out to a human face

  ✽ become orientated to their main carer(s), and look at their face when feeding

  ✽ begin to connect what they hear with what they see

  ✽ are able to show an increasingly wide range of feelings and responses including pleasure, fear, excitement, contentment, unhappiness

  ✽ have some awareness of the feeling and emotions of others.

Social and Emotional Development at 6 Months

Development during the first six months is very rapid. If babies have been stimulated by the presence of others during those periods they will show great interest in their environment and respond happily to positive attention.

Around this stage babies:

* show a marked preference for their main carer(s)
* reach out for familiar people and show a desire to be picked up and held
* begin to be more reserved with or afraid of strangers
* show a range of emotions including anger and pleasure through body movements, facial expression and vocally
* smile at their own image in the mirror
* may like to play peek-a-boo
* play alone with contentment
* stop crying when communicated with
* become more aware of themselves in relation to other people and things.

Around 6 months babies may also have the following skills:

* Look at their hands and feet with interest
* Drink from a cup that is held for them
* Have increasing use of their hands to hold things.

Social and Emotional Development at 9 Months

By this age, babies will have formed strong attachments with their main carer(s) Babies take great pleasure in playing with their carer and learn a great deal from this interaction.

At this stage babies:

* clearly distinguish familiar people and show a marked preference for them
* show a fear of strangers and need reassurance when in their company, often clinging to the known adult
* play peek-a-boo, copy hand clapping and pat a mirror image
* still cry for attention to their needs, but will also use their voice to attract people
* show pleasure and interest at familiar words
* understand 'No'

* begin to respond to their own name
* try to copy sounds
* show signs of willingness to wait for attention
* offer objects but do not release them.

Around 9 months babies may:

* put their hands around a cup or bottle when feeding.

Social and Emotional Development at 12 Months

By this age, many babies will have started to stand independently and possibly walk. This enables them to gain a completely different view of the world and they are able to explore their environment.

At around this age babies:

* like to be within sight or hearing of a familiar adult
* can distinguish between different members of the family and act socially with them
* will wave goodbye
* may be shy with strangers
* are capable of expressing a variety of emotional responses including anger, fear, happiness and humour
* become increasingly aware of the emotions of others
* actively seek attention by vocalising rather than crying
* copy the actions and sounds of adults or children
* will obey simple instructions
* know their own name.

Around 12 months they may have the following skills:

* Assist with feeding themselves by holding a spoon and may drink from a cup by them
* Help with dressing by holding out their arms or legs.

Social and Emotional Development at 15 Months

At this age toddlers use their main carer as a safe base from which to explore the world. They are anxious and apprehensive about being physically separated from them.

Around this age toddlers:

❋ have a sense of 'me' and 'mine' and begin to express them defiantly

❋ can point to members of the family in answer to questions ('where's granny?)

❋ tend to show off

❋ show interest in other children

❋ show jealousy of the attention given by adults to other children

❋ are emotionally changeable

❋ are not dissuaded from undesirable behaviour by verbal reasoning

❋ throw toys or objects when angry

❋ resist changes in routine

❋ swing from dependence to wanting to be independent.

Around 15 months they may have the following skills:

❋ Hold a cup and drink without assistance

❋ Hold a spoon and bring it to the mouth

❋ Help with dressing and undressing.

Social and Emotional Development at 18 Months

At this age children are very egocentric. They can often be defiant and resistant at this age in an attempt to protect themselves and their individuality, having only recently discovered themselves as separate individuals.

At this stage children:

❋ are trying to establish themselves as members of the social group

❋ begin to understand the things that adults think are important and begin to believe and behave similarly

❋ are still very dependent on a familiar carer and often return to a fear of strangers

❋ respond to stopping doing something when the word 'No' is used (often needs reinforcing)

❋ tend to follow their main carer(s) around, be sociable and imitate them by helping with small household tasks

❋ are conscious of their family group

❋ imitate and mimic others during their play; engage in solitary or parallel play

❋ show intense curiosity

❋ show some social emotions, for example show sympathy for someone who is hurt

❋ cannot tolerate frustration

❋ have intense mood swings, from dependence to independence, eagerness to irritation, co-operation to resistance.

Around 18 months they may have the following skills:

❋ Use a cup and spoon well

❋ Take off an item of clothing and help with dressing themselves although still in nappies, can make their carer aware of their toileting needs through words or restless behaviour.

Bonding and Attachment

An infant's social and emotional development is significantly influenced by the early relationships they experience in life. A 'bond of attachment' is a term used to describe an affectionate two-way relationship that develops between an infant and an adult. It refers to the process by which a loving, lasting bond is formed between a baby and a key person or persons in a baby's life.

Experiencing a bond of attachment is essential to children's healthy social and emotional development. When a bond has been established an infant will try to stay close to that adult and will appear to want to be cared for by them. By the end of a first year, an infant will exhibit a marked preference for that person with whom they have formed an attachment and may show stranger anxiety and separation distress.

There are basic biological reasons for attachment; babies are vulnerable and need protection. They will instinctively seek out someone to protect them and become attached to that person and will try to ensure close contact, especially in time of distress. The bonding may be largely physical, but may also be maintained by sound, or by sight.

The other consideration is the biological need in adults to look after their babies, to cuddle, comfort and keep them safe. A bond of attachment is established over a period of time, can be divided into four main stages:

❋ during pregnancy

❋ at delivery

❋ immediately after delivery

❋ during the first six months.

By the end of the first six months of life, babies will usually have established a bond of attachment, and their experiences during this period are crucial.

The interaction between the babies and its carers is significant and focuses on carers meeting the baby's needs.

Positive feedback from the baby to the carer will also strengthen the bond. For example, the baby expresses needs by crying, smiling, babbling, clinging or raising their arms. The carer meets the baby's needs by feeding, talking, cuddling the baby. Gradually the baby learns to trusts that the carer will meet their needs and the bond is established.

Upon initiating positive interaction, the bond may be further strengthened. The carer, for instance, initiates positive interaction by talking to the baby; the baby responds positively by cooing or smiling. The carer is then motivated to initiate further positive interaction and the cycle continues. This leads to feelings of self-esteem and self-worth on the part of the carer and strengthens the bond.

Bonds of attachment are important as they affect all aspects of a child's development. A strong bond of attachment helps to motivate the carer to meet their children's physical needs and if the baby is responsive the carers' self-esteem will be increased.

Children who have a strong bond of attachment will have the confidence to explore and make discoveries and are therefore more likely to learn as they feel able to leave their carers and explore. A bond of attachment will motivate a carer and baby to engage in early conversations that encourage the development of language.

If babies have their emotional needs met through the attachment relationship, they will be more able to cope with stress and frustration.

In terms of emotional development a child learns to be independent through experiencing dependence. Another important result of a strong bond is the development of a positive self-image. Children learn to understand themselves through the responses and reactions of those close to them. If the messages they receive are largely positive, they will help to build self-esteem and a positive self-image.

Children with a positive self-image will be able to tolerate frustration more easily, they will be easier to manage, control or discipline. Children with a strong bond of attachment are better able to cope with fears and worries, as they feel safe and trust their carer to care for them and protect them from overwhelming fears and anxieties. A strong bond of attachment helps develop children's feelings of trust in their carer and their sense of security. This helps children to feel safe and encourages them to rely on other people.

This is essential to the development of any relationship and through the development of a bond of attachment; they learn to take party in a reciprocal relationship.

Around 18 months, children with a strong bond of attachment will show social emotions. They may show empathy or understanding of how other people feel. They may show care for others, sympathy, pride and embarrassment.

Through experiencing embarrassment, children can experience shame and guilt, and in the right balance this can be a healthy way to develop a conscience and learn right from wrong. Without a conscience a child's behaviour may be totally self-centred.

Attachment Behaviour Patterns

Up to 3 to 4 months, babies generally do not mind who is with them (an exception may be very hungry breast-fed babies).

At 3 to 5 months babies start to decide who they feel safe with.

At around 6 to 7 months babies will express their preference clearly and will show anxiety in the company of strangers. The response will be more marked if the baby is not being held and reassured by the person with whom they have formed an attachment, and it is in a strange place.

At 8 to 18 months babies will start to make additional attachments if other adults are willing.

From two years onwards anxiety and separation distress slowly start to disappear in well-attached children so long as the separation is not for too long.

Language Development

Both parents and their babies are active participants in early conversations. If early gazing is met with a smile and coos and gurgles are noticed and imitated, then an atmosphere is established in which a baby can develop a language of words.

Babies' language skills develop through a series of identifiable stages.

How language develops from birth to 18 months (as with all development charts mentioning ages, these should be seen as a rough developmental guide).

Baby's Age	Baby's Understanding	Baby's Expressions	Carer's Response
0–1 month	Responds to sounds, especially familiar voices; goes quiet when picked up; establishes feeding rhythms and patterns	Signs of intentional communication: eye contact; crying, grunting, sighing; blowing bubbles or raspberries; feeding rhythms develop as 'cues' for carer to respond to, for example breaking off gaze when less hungry	Picking baby up, talking face-to-face, responding to baby's cues whilst feeding by talking, smiling or staying silent
1–4 months	First smile in response to approaches and talking; recognition of main carer(s) and familiar faces and objects (e.g. bottle); anticipation of being picked up (excited limb movements)	Non-crying noises (cooing and gurgling); first begins to laugh; cries become more expressive of needs (hunger, tiredness, impatience etc)	Learning to distinguish cries and respond to them differently; imitating baby's sounds to encourage repetition
4–6 months	Recognises and responds to familiar sounds, voices and objects; reacts to tones in voices (will become upset by anger and will be cheered by happiness); begins to enjoy music and rhymes, particularly if accompanied by actions	Babble talk begins; makes noises to show feeling of pleasure or distress	Talking in response to baby's noises and daily experiences
6–9 months	Understanding signs (e.g. bib means food); understanding of 'up' and 'down'; responds to own name and other familiar names; continues to enjoy music and rhymes and will now attempt to join in with actions	Makes appropriate gestures, such as raising arms to be picked up; continuation of babbling, tries out a few single syllables; can imitate, clap and play peek-a-boo	Tailoring speech to understanding using clear simple words to assist learning games; talking as baby does things

Age	Understanding	Expression	Response
9–12 months	Understanding of games like dropping and picking up a toy; understands 'No'; follows simple instructions; enjoys songs, action rhythms; understands own daily routine	May produce first words 'dad' or 'mama'; much expressive babbling; babbling begins to reflect the intonation of speech; playing with toys and objects to show they know what they are for	Designing speech to respond to baby (naming things repeatedly); giving instructions; asking questions
12–15 months	Follows simple commands; can point to pictures and known objects; knows parts of the body; listens carefully to carer(s) and others; laughs at humorous events (e.g. funny faces)	May say two or three words, but still much speech-like chatter; shows the use of things by more complex play; pointing accompanied by a single word is the basis for communication	Echoing baby's words; pointing out new words; questions; commands; basing conversations on recent events
15–20 months	Recognises many objects and pictures of objects; can make plans and anticipate future; begins to understand 'in' and 'on' and 'me' and 'her'; understands things and events in own daily life	Single word vocabulary continues to increase and will include words such as 'more', 'all gone', 'no', as well as some verbs, object names; attempts to copy sounds such as car and animal noises; may use vocabulary for requesting and commenting ('Mummy gone' 'Coat on'); vocabulary increases between around 10 to 30 words; there can be a wide range in expression ability at this time	Many occasions for conversations through play, outings, shared activities
20–24 months	Understands longer sentences, recognises objects and pictures in greater numbers; can match familiar objects; understands 'more', 'here' and 'now'; will enjoy and follow very simple stories	Vocabulary increasing from 30 to 60 or 70 words, some joined up to make two-word sentences; makes up own words, tries to tell you about things that have happened	More to listen to, as baby starts talking more and initiating conversations; may have to interpret words

Cognitive Development

Cognitive development is the way in which babies and children process their everyday experiences and build up an understanding of the world.

From birth to two years the stage of cognitive development is known as **Sensory–motor development**.

At this stage, the child will:

❋ learn principally through **sight** and **touch** and through **movement**

❋ process information **visually** as **images**

❋ become aware that objects continue to exist when not in view (known as **object permanence**). This awareness develops around 8 to 12 months

❋ use abilities intelligently and begin to learn through trial and error

❋ be **egocentric**, that is they can only see the world from their own point of view.

Questions for **R**eview

1. i) State the typical postures of a baby at the following ages

    ii) State how the postures at this age may affect positioning of the baby for massage

    a) 1-month-old baby

    _____

    _____

    _____

    _____

    _____

    _____

    _____

    _____

    b) 3-month-old baby

    _____

    _____

    _____

    _____

    _____

    _____

    _____

    c) 6-month-old baby

    _____

    _____

    _____

    _____

    _____

    _____

    _____

d) 9-month-old baby

_____
_____
_____
_____
_____
_____
_____

2. Briefly describe the social and emotional development of a baby at the following ages:

   i) 1 month

   _____
   _____
   _____
   _____
   _____

   ii) 3 months

   _____
   _____
   _____
   _____
   _____

   iii) 12 months

   _____
   _____
   _____
   _____
   _____

iv) 18 months

_____

_____

_____

_____

_____

_____

3. What is meant by a 'bond of attachment'?

_____

_____

_____

_____

_____

_____

4. By what age do babies usually form a bond of attachment with their main carer(s)?

_____

_____

_____

_____

_____

5. State three reasons why bonds of attachment are important for babies and their parents/carer.

_____

_____

_____

_____

6.   At what age does a baby generally:

   i) First smile in response to talking?

   _____

   _____

   ii) Establish feeding rhythms as cues for their carer to respond to?

   _____

   _____

   iii) Begin babble talk?

   _____

   _____

7.   What is meant by cognitive development in babies?

   _____

   _____

   _____

   _____

8.   State three principal ways in which babies learn from birth to two years

   _____

   _____

   _____

   _____

06 Consultation and Record Keeping for Baby Massage

Consultation and Record Keeping for Baby Massage

Good communication skills are essential for creating a positive, trusting and co-operative relationship between a baby massage instructor and a parent/carer.

A good instructor will have a calm and relaxed manner, whilst being friendly and approachable, and be able to put parents at their ease.

It is important for instructors to consider that this is a new experience for parents as well as their babies, and the more relaxed they feel the more positive the experience will be for all concerned. A good instructor will also be supportive of parents and non-judgmental of their parenting styles. It is important to consider that parents may be feeling stressed and tired themselves, and need to feel that the instructor can identify with their experiences and show empathy, whilst at the same time give positive encouragement as to how massage can help their babies and themselves.

It is important to ensure that the environment in which the consultation is to take place is as comfortable, private and warm as possible. If parents feel relaxed they are more likely to communicate more openly and it will be easier for an instructor to establish a rapport and help identify their needs.

By the end of this chapter you will be able to relate the following knowledge to your role as an instructor/parent or carer:

* the reasons for a consultation before a baby massage session
* the communication skills required for a successful session
* the contra-indications to baby massage
* the reasons why medical referral and advice may be needed before baby massage
* the ethics concerned with baby massage provision
* legislation relevant to a baby massage instructor.

A consultation is essential before carrying out the instruction session in order that the instructor may:

✻ familiarise themselves with the baby and its parents or carers

✻ help put the parent/carer at ease, answer any queries and allay their fears about the instruction session

✻ help identify the baby's medical history and to establish their current state of health

✻ check whether there are any contra-indications and whether the parent should be advised to seek the GP's advice before massaging

✻ identify a parent's needs, desires and expectations (parents may need advice on massage to help with sleeping problems, colic etc)

✻ explain the benefits of baby massage for the baby and its parents/carers

✻ determine the need for special care or adaptation of treatment, such as in the case of a special needs baby

✻ outline and explain the format of the massage instruction session.

Client Communication Skills

When exchanging information during a consultation, there are four main types of communication skills:

✻ verbal communication

✻ listening skills

✻ non-verbal communication

✻ written communication.

Verbal Communication

During a consultation for baby massage instruction, it is important for the instructor to realise that a parent's attention can be diverted due to their baby's presence. An instructor will therefore need to be patient and flexible in their approach.

Parents will like to feel that the instructor is able to identify with their needs and that they have been listened to. When speaking to a parent, it is important to choose words which convey intent clearly, concisely and tactfully and to avoid using language the parent may not understand, such as medical terminology.

Verbal communication involves co-operation from both the parent and the instructor and when exchanging information there should be a period of reflective pause in the conversation periodically, in order to verify the message intended, and give an opportunity for any corrections or alterations to be made.

Listening Skills

One of the most important skills in verbal communication is the art of listening, and through effective listening an instructor can identify with the parent's/baby's needs and devise an instruction session accordingly.

Therapists should be aware that parents may not always make themselves understood and they may be speaking through a screen of emotionally charged feelings. Effective listening will therefore involve understanding not only what the parent is trying to say, but the tone and the emotion with which the information is imparted.

Active listening should always be undertaken in a non-judgmental way, which will help the parent to feel safe to disclose sensitive and personal information in an honest and open way. Part of being non- judgmental involves an instructor withholding their own personal evaluation and thoughts on the parent's situation and respecting a parent's right to reveal their feelings in a supported environment.

It is important for therapists to realise that parents may be guarded about disclosing personal feelings until there is an established measure of trust between them.

Instructors need to take care to consider their attitude and body language when carrying out a consultation, and the importance of maintaining eye contact.

Non-verbal Communication

In order to enhance communication with parents, instructors need to consider the implications of non-verbal communication: messages that are projected by the body without the speaker's awareness.

Non-verbal messages are an important part of communication as they will often convey information about the emotional state of the parent.

Non-verbal signs may include:

Facial expressions—lack of eye contact, frowning, grimacing

Gestures—gripping the sides of the chair, fidgeting, nodding, making fists

Sounds—sighs, grunts and groans, changes in breath, yawning

Posture—hunched shoulders.

Written Communication

Baby consultation forms and instruction records are necessary as they help the instructor to form a structure for the consultation, and may be used as a guide to ensure nothing is overlooked. For ethical reasons it is essential that the parent/guardian consent to the instruction by signing the consultation form and the treatment record.

An example of a baby massage consultation form and instruction record is illustrated on pages 113–117.

Confidentiality

Confidentiality is an important part of the professional relationship between an instructor and a parent.

Whilst carrying out a consultation it is important for an instructor to stress that all personal information recorded relating to the baby/parents will remain completely confidential, and that information will not be disclosed to a third party without the parent's written consent.

Maintaining confidentiality will help establish a good rapport with the parent and encourage their confidence in the instructor.

Instructors can maintain confidentiality by:

* carrying out the consultation in as private an area as possible
* ensuring that all baby consultation and treatment records are stored in a secure place
* ensuring that baby records and personal details are never left lying around
* never discussing a baby's/parents personal details or their treatment with another person, unless it is to liaise with another professional concerned with the parent's progress, and the parent's permission has been granted.

Contra-indications to Baby Massage

It is essential that before carrying out a baby massage instruction session that possible contra-indications are discussed with the parents or carers.

The parent or carer needs to be advised of when it may not be possible to massage their baby and why.

Baby massage should ideally begin after the baby has had a six- to eight-week medical check with their GP. However, premature babies may be gently massaged with prior consultation with the GP/hospital although the massage may consist of mainly stroking at the initial stages.

The ideal time for massage is when the baby is not too tired or hungry. It is best to advise the parents that the baby should be fed approximately one to one-and-a-half hours before the massage session begins.

It is important for the instructor to advise the parents to respect the baby's needs by not massaging when the baby is sleeping or crying.

It is also important to advise parents to seek professional help if their baby is unwell. Parents are invariably the best judges as to when their baby is not well and will realise that the baby will probably not wish to be massaged, but may wish to be comforted and held.

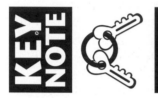

Parents should also be encouraged to ask permission from the baby before beginning to massage, by observing verbal and non-verbal signs from the baby and if the baby is unresponsive to try again at a later stage.

Conditions that are contra-indicated to baby massage include:

Infectious Diseases—parents should be advised that their baby should never be massaged whilst suffering from an infectious disease to avoid spreading the infection. Babies should never be massaged if suffering from a fever.

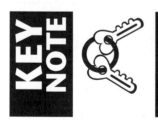

All babies are liable to infection. They have delicate skin and mucous membranes which means bacteria can readily gain access to the body. It is also important to consider that a baby's defence mechanisms against infection are under-developed in the first months of life.

Contagious Skin Disorders—in the case of contagious skin disorders, massage presents the risk of further aggravating the tissues and should therefore be avoided. There is also the risk of cross infection. Conditions such as impetigo and ringworm are amongst the most common childhood skin infections encountered.

Recent Fractures, Sprains and Swelling—parents should be advised to avoid massaging a fracture, sprain or swelling until all signs of inflammation and injury have healed. Massaging over the site of an unstable fracture may hinder the healing process and could cause internal complications.

Recent haemorrhage—in the case of a recent haemorrhage, massage should be avoided due to the stimulation of circulation and the risk of internal or external bleeding. Parents should be advised to seek medical advice.

Jaundice—is a symptom of gall bladder or liver dysfunction that occurs when there is an excess of bilirubin causing the skin, eyes and mucous membranes to appear yellow. Massage should be avoided until the liver is fully functional.

Meningitis—is an acute inflammation of the membranes that cover the brain and spinal cord and requires immediate medical treatment. Meningitis most frequently results from an infection, either bacterial or viral.

Viral meningitis occurs most commonly after mumps, but is not as serious as bacterial meningitis.

Bacterial meningitis is serious, but can be treated with antibiotics if it is diagnosed early enough; the symptoms of meningitis are a fever, stiff neck, lethargy, headaches, drowsiness and intolerance to bright lights. In some cases there may be a purple-red rash.

Meningitis can be difficult to detect in babies and small children, whose inability to communicate what they are feeling may lead to a delay in diagnosis.

In babies suffering from meningitis under the age of two, the fontanelle will bulge slightly. Massage is therefore contra-indicated until all signs of infection have passed.

Childhood Leukaemia—is a malignant disease of the bone marrow cells that form white blood cells.

In leukaemia the bone marrow produces many abnormal white blood cells (leukaemic cells), and a reduced number of normal white cells, red cells and platelets. The leukaemic cells infiltrate the liver, spleen and lymph glands.

The main form of leukaemia in childhood is acute lymphoblastic leukaemia, and may produce the following symptoms: pale skin, pink or purple spots on the skin, easily bruised skin, lack of energy, swollen lymph nodes in the neck, armpits and groin, fever, pain in the limb bones and joints, bleeding gums.

Leukaemia requires medical treatment and massage would be contra-indicated. It is important to remember that as drug treatment increases susceptibility to infection, children or babies with leukaemia should be kept away from anyone with an infection.

Consultation with the child's oncologist is necessary before providing any form of massage.

Osteoporosis/brittle bones—in any condition where there is decrease in bone density the bones become brittle and are liable to fracture easily. Massage is therefore contra-indicated in the presence of osteoporosis or any condition that presents brittle bones.

Conditions that may be contra-indicated to baby massage or may require GP referral and an adaptation of treatment include:

Recent operation/surgery—always advise the parent to consult the baby's GP and/or Surgeon before massaging their baby post-operatively. Generally, massage should not be given on or near the area for at least six to eight weeks after surgery. Breaks or openings in the scars or sutures should not be massaged, as it could disrupt the healing process or cause infections. If endorsed by the baby's physician, massage to other areas may be beneficial.

In many cases, once a child has recovered from the surgery, massage can be soothing to both parent and baby and can help parents to overcome any anxiety they may have over handling their baby in a fragile state.

Congenital heart condition—it is essential to take a detailed history of the baby's heart condition along with the details of any surgical /medical treatment that has been carried out.

The most common forms of congenital heart defects are:

Aortic valve stenosis—this refers to a narrowing (stenosis) of the aortic valve of the heart that gives rise to a heart murmur.

If the narrowing is sufficient to obstruct the flow of blood, the heart has to work harder than usual. This does not usually cause problems in childhood but may give rise to heart strain in adulthood, so an operation is often recommended if the narrowing is severe. Many children with mild aortic stenosis do not require treatment.

Atrial septal defect—this is a form of congenital heart disease in which there is a hole between the left and right atria, the upper chambers of the heart; some blood passes through this hole. The right ventricle, one of the two lower chambers of the heart, has to pump this extra blood around the lungs. With time this can put a strain on the heart and an operation to close the defect during childhood may be recommended.

Pulmonary valve stenosis—a congenital lesion of the heart, in which there is narrowing (stenosis) of the pulmonary valve at the exit of the right ventricle, which may obstruct the flow of blood. The narrowing of the valve gives rise to a heart murmur which enables the diagnosis to be made. If there is an obstruction which may impose strain on the heart, an operation to relieve the narrowing may be recommended.

Ventricular septal defect—this is a form of congenital heart disease in which there is a hole in the septum or partition between the rights and left ventricles, the lower chambers of the heart: the hole that allows blood to flow from left to right. As a consequence the heart works harder than usual as extra blood gets pumped to the lungs unnecessarily. Sometimes the septal defect is so large that the baby becomes breathless and is unable to feed properly, in which case surgical treatment is needed.

If the defect is large and does not close an operation may be needed.

Transposition of the Great Vessels—is a severe heart abnormality in which the aorta, the main artery, rises from the right ventricle, one of the lower chambers of the heart), and the pulmonary artery from the left ventricle, instead of the other way round. The baby will appear blue due to there being very little oxygen in the blood circulating around the body. Babies affected by this condition need urgent medical treatment and a surgical intervention to correct the flow of blood.

When proposing to use massage for a child with a cardiac or circulatory condition, the baby's physician must provide advice and approval in order to rule out any potential risk. A baby or small child's circulatory system may be unable to accommodate the increased flow of blood through the heart provided by the massage.

Not all cardiac conditions are contra-indicated for massage. However, it is essential for the instructor to consult the baby's physician before advising the parent to proceed with any form of massage.

In general, gentle massage and relaxed hand placements may be helpful due to the relaxation effect, but duration and frequency would need to be decided on an individual basis, depending on the baby's condition and medical advice offered at the time of the proposed treatment.

Congenital dislocation of the hip—in this condition the hip joint is unstable because of the failure to develop properly at birth. It may be associated with the position of the foetus in the uterus, but there may also be a genetic link.

When the hip is dislocated, the head of the femur may become displaced from the socket in the pelvis and if left untreated will affect the development of walking.

It is important that the baby's hips are tested soon after birth and then at regular intervals up to one year. The baby's legs are held in the abducted position by the use of splints. A typical click can be felt as the dislocated head of the femur slips back into its socket.

Massage and any form of manipulation (such as stretching) is contra-indicated for congenital dislocated hips as it may interfere with the healing process and may cause the baby discomfort.

Spastic conditions—in spastic conditions there is generally an increase in muscle tone which can result in rigidity. In the case of a baby with a spastic condition, it is important to remember that growth is actively occurring all the time and that massage may help to increase joint mobility and reduce rigidity, as well as offer comfort and support.

Always encourage parents to refer to the baby's GP concerning the nature of the spastic condition.

Dysfunction of the nervous system—this is an umbrella term for disorders of neurological origin. Any dysfunction of the nervous system should be discussed with the GP prior to massage.

Epilepsy—epilepsy is a condition in which there are recurrent attacks of temporary disturbance of brain function. Epilepsy is a complex condition and may take many different forms. The condition will vary with each child and symptoms may range from disturbances in consciousness that are hardly noticeable to mild sensations and lapses of concentration to severe seizures with convulsions.

Always advise the parent to seek GP's advice in all cases before proceeding with massage.

If massage is advised, keep the sessions brief and monitor the results carefully (i.e. note whether there is any increase in seizure activity during or after massage).

Asthma—childhood asthma is common and symptoms include wheezing, coughing, increased mucus production, rapid, shallow or laboured breathing and prolonged expiration.

Massage is contra-indicated during an acute attack; however, massage may be helpful in the sub-acute stage to help reduce anxiety.

Conditions that may present as a localised contra-indication and restrict treatment include:

Recent Immunisation—it is best to advise parents to wait at least 48 hours to see how the immunisation will affect their baby. (The polio vaccination can, for instance, produce a reaction as a result of the live vaccine.)

If the baby has no reaction to the vaccination then the injection site may be treated as a localised contra-indication and after a week may be massaged to help disperse any lump that may be left.

Skin Disorders—a baby's skin is very sensitive and delicate and therefore any inflammation may be exacerbated by massage. Babies often develop rashes and affected areas should be avoided.

Inflammatory Skin Conditions—the decision as to whether a baby with eczema and psoriasis may be massaged will be determined by the condition and the cause of the inflammation present. Massage is usually helpful if eczema is dry and flaky and the skin is unbroken, however massage would be contra-indicated if the inflammation has lesions which may be spread.

Skin allergies—if a parent indicates that a baby has had a previous reaction to oils or lotions, note these on the baby's massage records.

To determine sensitivity of a lubricant a simple patch test should be carried out by placing a small amount of the oil or lotion on an area such as the wrist and waiting for 30 minutes to determine tolerance.

Cuts and Bruises—parents should be advised to treat cuts and bruises as localised contra-indications and avoid the affected area to avoid discomfort.

Unhealed navel—no massage should be carried out around this area until it is healed.

A note for Instructors and Parents

Caution Sites

Instructors and parents need to be aware of areas of their baby's body that warrant caution, as deep pressure over the area may cause damage to underlying structures, such as blood vessels, nerves, organs and lymph nodes.

It is necessary for parents to be advised of the following areas by instructors in order that they avoid using strong pressure in massage that may cause discomfort or damage to their baby:

* front of the neck and throat
* orbital (eyes)
* back of the neck
* over the spinous processes of the spine
* under the arm (the axilla)
* brachial region of the upper arm (middle aspect of the upper arm)
* front of the elbow (cubital region)
* back of the elbow
* mid-back, kidney area (upper lumbar area)
* umbilical area (navel)
* inner aspect of upper leg (femoral triangle)
* back of knee (popliteal fossa)
* groin area (inguinal area).

A Baby Massage Consultation Form

Confidential

Baby's Name: _____ Date of Birth: _____

Parent/Carer's Name: _____

Address: _____

_____

Tel no: _____ Daytime_____ Evening

Has your baby had his/her paediatric check? Yes ( ) No ( )

Results/Comments: _____

_____

Doctor's Name: _____ Surgery: _____

Health Visitor: _____

Birth details

Type/Weight: _____

Additional information: _____

_____

Weekly weight gain

above average ( )   average ( )   below average ( )

Sleep pattern

good ( )   normal ( )   poor ( )

Eating/feeding

good ( )   normal ( )   poor ( )

Parental/Guardian Note

The following information is needed for safety reasons before proceeding with the massage instruction. There may be certain reasons when it may not be possible for you to massage your baby and you may need to refer to your GP before proceeding.

Do any of the following apply to your baby?

Dates and Details

	Y	N	
Recent operation/surgery?	[ ]	[ ]	_____
Current medical treatment?	[ ]	[ ]	_____
Recent immunisation?	[ ]	[ ]	_____
Skin disorder?	[ ]	[ ]	_____
Recent haemorrhage?	[ ]	[ ]	_____
Recent fracture or sprain?	[ ]	[ ]	_____
Cuts, abrasions or skin rashes?	[ ]	[ ]	_____
Allergies?	[ ]	[ ]	_____
Any dysfunction of the nervous system?	[ ]	[ ]	_____
Spastic condition?	[ ]	[ ]	_____
Any recent or current infections?	[ ]	[ ]	_____

Are there any other conditions relevant to your baby that have not been mentioned above?

Details: _____

_____

Parental/Guardian's Consent

I give my consent to receive baby massage instruction from _____

I understand all information recorded concerning my baby will be held as strictly confidential.

Parent's/Guardian's signature: _____ Date: _____

Record of Baby Massage Instruction

Session No 1

Date of session: _____ Name of instructor: _____

Type of massage sequence instructed: _____

Oils used: _____

Results/baby's response to massage: _____

_____

_____

After care advice given: _____

_____

Parent/Guardian signature: _____

Instructor's signature: _____

Session No 2

Feedback from last session: _____

_____

_____

Date of session: _____ Name of instructor: _____

Type of massage sequence instructed: _____

Oils used: _____

Results/baby's response to massage: _____

_____

_____

After care advice given: _____

_____

Parent/Guardian signature: _____

Instructor's signature: _____

Session No 3

Feedback from last session: _____

_____

_____

Date of session: _____ Name of instructor: _____

Type of massage sequence instructed: _____

Oils used: _____

Results/baby's response to massage: _____

_____

_____

After care advice given: _____

_____

Parent/Guardian signature: _____

Instructor's signature: _____

Session No 4

Feedback from last session: _____

_____

_____

Date of session: _____ Name of instructor: _____

Type of massage sequence instructed: _____

Oils used: _____

Results/baby's response to massage: _____

_____

_____

After care advice given: _____

_____

Parent/Guardian signature: _____

Instructor's signature: _____

Baby Massage Instruction Parental Feedback Form

Please complete this evaluation form to help your Baby Massage Instructor ensure that you have received all relevant information necessary.

Baby's Name: _____

Parent/Guardian: _____

Instructor: _____

Were all the instructions you received clear, concise and informative?

Yes   (   )   No   (   )

Comments _____

Were you given sufficient time to ask questions?

Yes   (   )   No   (   )

Comments _____

Did you fully understand how to massage your baby using the relevant massage strokes?

Yes   (   )   No   (   )

Comments _____

Are there any areas which you are unsure about?

Yes   (   )   No   (   )

Comments _____

How do you feel about massaging your baby? _____

_____

_____

Please indicate your experience of learning baby massage.

	Low									High
Enjoyable	1	2	3	4	5	6	7	8	9	10
Helpful	1	2	3	4	5	6	7	8	9	10
Interesting	1	2	3	4	5	6	7	8	9	10

Do you have any other comments? _____

_____

_____

Signed:_____ Parent/Guardian

Date:_____

Ethics associated with baby massage provision

As a baby massage instructor, it is important to recognise that babies are aware human beings who deserve respect, tenderness and warmth.

The baby's and parent's consent should always be sought prior to the massage instruction session.

The parent may consent by signing the consultation and treatment record and the baby's consent may be offered by their verbal or non-verbal cues to their parent/guardian or to the instructor.

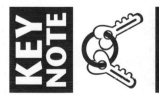

KEY NOTE

A code of ethics for Baby Massage Instructors must take account of the fact that a baby has the same rights as an adult, although they are represented by their parent or guardian.

Legislation Associated with Baby Massage Instruction

Baby massage instructors need to be aware of legislation that is relevant to their role; in particular the Children's Act, Health and Safety at Work Act, along with any Local Authority Bye-Laws in the area(s) in which they are instructing.

The Children's Act 1989

The Children's Act of 1989 came into effect in 1991. It is an important piece of legislation concerning children and the way they are treated.

The Children's Act gives children rights in that they should be consulted, listened to, protected and given their chance to voice their feelings and opinions.

Most importantly, the Children's Act has given children a voice in that it recognises that they should be treated with respect, and as an individual.

As baby massage instruction is a service provided to families, it is important to be aware of this legislation, as babies and children have the same rights as adults.

Parental consent should therefore always be obtained prior to the massage session, along with the consent of the baby itself.

The key points of the Children's Act are as follows:

* Children's welfare in both private and public sectors is made a priority
* Recognition that children are best brought up within their families, wherever possible
* Aims to prevent unwarranted interference in family life
* Requires local authorities to provide services for children and families in need
* Promotes partnership between children, parents and local authorities
* Improves the way that courts deal with children and families
* Gives right of appeal against court decisions
* Protects the rights of parents with children being looked after by local authorities
* Aims to ensure children looked after by local authorities are provided with a good standard of care

Although unpleasant to contemplate, there are several forms of abuse that children can be submitted to and these may include physical injury, neglect, emotional ill treatment or sexual abuse.

As the nature of baby massage instruction involves babies being unclothed, signs of physical abuse may be evident. A therapist may also be aware of behavioural indications.

If a therapist was concerned for the safety and welfare of a child, they would have a moral duty to take appropriate action if possible violation of the Children's Act was witnessed or suspected.

It is essential however, that therapists carefully consider their responsibilities to the children and their family, and avoid acting irresponsibly.

It may be appropriate, if genuinely concerned, and it is not possible to gain the trust of the parents, to speak confidentiality with the child's GP or health visitor.

Guidelines on Code of Ethics for Baby Massage Instruction

❋ Always carry out a consultation with the parent or carer to ensure the baby is suitable for massage.

❋ Always advise the parent or carer to seek medical advice if the baby is under medical care.

❋ Ensure that the baby and its parent consent fully to the massage instruction.

❋ Never abuse the relationship between yourself, the parent/guardian or the baby.

❋ Never give unqualified advice, and use your skills of instruction within the limitations of the therapy and training you have undertaken.

❋ Ensure that you respect the baby's and the parent's or guardian's wishes at all times throughout the instruction session, irrespective of their race, creed, colour, sex or religious views.

❋ Ensure that the working environment provided for the baby massage instruction complies with current health, safety and hygiene legislation.

❋ Keep accurate, up-to-date and confidential records of treatment and instruction provided.

❋ Be adequately insured to practise the massage instruction through a professional association.

❋ Always conduct yourself in a professional manner and be courteous to the baby and its parent or guardian at all times.

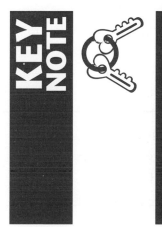

KEY NOTE

An Important Note for Instructors

The Criminal Records Bureau has now made it a requirement for Baby Massage Instructors to obtain a **Standard Disclosure Certificate** if they wish to provide Baby Massage Instruction (this does not apply to health care practitioners who have already been through this process in their profession).

For details, information and the procedures for obtaining a Standard Disclosure Certificate, the Criminal Records Bureau should be contacted on **0870 9090 811**.

Other Legislation Relevant to Baby Massage Instructors

There are a number of pieces of legislation that are of importance to a baby massage instructor and these need to be taken account of, regardless of where the instruction takes place (for instance if using a community centre for classes check out local bye-laws, health and safety, fire precautions first).

Health and Safety at Work Act 1974

The Health and Safety at Work Act provides a comprehensive legal framework to promote and encourage high standards of health and safety in the workplace.

The Health and Safety at Work Act covers a range of legislation relating to health and safety and both the employer and employee have responsibilities under the Act.

If there are more than five employees a written Health and Safety Policy is required.

The Responsibilities of the Employer

❋ Safeguard as far as possible the health, safety and welfare of themselves, their employees, contractors employees and members of the public.

❋ Keep all equipment up to health and safety standards.

❋ Have safety equipment checked regularly.

❋ Ensure the environment is free from toxic fumes.

❋ Ensure that all staff are aware of safety procedures, by providing safety information and training.

❋ Ensure safe systems of work.

The Responsibilities of the Employee

❋ Adhere to the workplace rules and regulations concerning safety.

❋ Follow safe working practices and attending training as required.

❋ Take reasonable care to avoid injury to themselves and others.

❋ Co-operate with others in all matters relating to health and safety.

❋ Not to interfere or wilfully misuse anything provided to protect their health and safety.

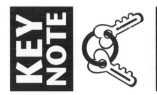

KEY NOTE

The Health and Safety Executive (HSE) have produced a guide to the laws on Health & Safety and it is a requirement that an employer displays a copy of this poster in the workplace.

Electricity at Work Regulations 1989

Regulations under this legislation are concerned with safety in connection the use of electricity.

It is recommended that electrical equipment be checked regularly (at least once a year) by a competent person such as a qualified electrician or the local electricity board.

All checks should be listed in a record book, stating the results of the tests and the recommendations and action taken in the case of defects.

In the case of legal action, a record book may serve as important evidence.

The checks that should be made in connection with electrical equipment include checking the fusing, insulation and that there are no loose or frayed wires.

Control of Substances Hazardous to Health (COSHH) 1998

Regulations under this legislation require employers to regulate employees' exposure to hazardous substances which may cause ill health or injury in the workplace and involves risk assessment.

Risk assessment involves making an itemised list of all the substances used in the workplace or sold to clients that may be hazardous to health. Attention is drawn to any substances which may cause irritation, cause allergic reactions, burn the skin, or give off fumes.

Instructions for handling and disposing of all hazardous substances must be made available to all staff and training provided, if required.

Manufacturers will usually supply information relating to their products and therapists should be able to recognise hazard warning symbols on labels and packaging.

Fire Precautions Act 1971

This legislation is concerned with fire prevention and adequate means of escape in the event of a fire.

The Act enforces that:

* all premises have fire-fighting equipment that is in good working order
* that the equipment is readily available and is suitable for all types of fire
* all staff are familiar with the establishment's evacuation procedures and the use of fire-fighting equipment
* fire escapes are kept free from obstruction and are clearly sign posted
* smoke alarms are fitted
* fire doors are fitted to help control the spread of fire.

It is a legal requirement for an employer to apply for a fire certificate if the business employs 20 or more staff.

It is important for all establishments to have set procedures in the event of a fire and that all staff is aware of it.

Fire Extinguishers

There are different fire extinguishers designed to deal with different types of fire.

From 1997, all fire extinguishers must be coloured red, but they all have different symbols and colour codes to show what type of fire they should be used for.

The main types of fire extinguishers are as follows:

* water (Red)
* CO_2 (Black)
* dry powder (Blue)
* foam (Cream).

The above fire extinguishers are coded in order to allow quick and easy identification and to avoid using the wrong type and put yourself and others in danger.

The main body colour of the extinguisher has changed over the past few years (any new extinguisher purchased or leased will be predominately red), however the type colours have remained the same.

NB. Any extinguishers that are not the correct colour will be replaced when they become unserviceable.

Water extinguishers are usually colour coded Red.

Other types of extinguishers fall into different categories, either:

* the entire body of the extinguisher is coloured in the type colour
* predominately red with a 5 per cent second colour to indicate the contents of the extinguisher
* predominately red with a bold coloured block in the relevant colour stating its type.

If you are in any doubt about the type of fire extinguisher to use in the workplace, it is advisable to contact your local Fire Safety Department for advice.

Health & Safety (First Aid) Regulation 1981

Under the Health and Safety (First-Aid) Regulations 1981 workplaces must have first-aid provision. The form it should take will depend on various factors including the nature and degree of hazards at work, what medical services are available and the number of employees.

The Health and Safety Executive (HSE) booklet **COP 42 first-aid at work (ISBN 0 11 885536 0)** contains an Approved Code of Practice and guidance notes to help employers meet their obligations.

The number of first-aiders needed in the workplace depends primarily on the degree of hazards. If the workplace is considered to be low-hazard (such as a holistic therapy clinic) there should be at least one first-aider for very 50 employees.

If there are fewer than 50 employees, there should always be an appointed person present when people are at work if no trained first-aider is available.

First-aiders must undertake training and obtain qualifications approved by the HSE. At present, first aid certificates are valid for three years. Refresher courses should be started before a certificate expires, otherwise a full course will need to be taken.

First-Aid Kits

First-aid kits should only contain items that a first-aider has been trained to use. They should always be adequately stocked and should **NOT** contain medication of any kind.

A general purpose first-aid kit will contain the following items: bandages, plasters wound dressings, antiseptic cream, quick sling, eye pads, scissors, safety pins and vinyl gloves.

First-aiders should record all cases they treat. Each record should include at least the name of the patient, date, place, time and circumstances of the accident and details of the injury and treatment given.

Reporting of Injuries, Diseases and Dangerous Occurrences Regulations 1985 (RIDDOR)

This legislation requires that all accidents which occur in the workplace, however minor, **MUST** be entered into an accident register. This is a requirement of the Health and Safety at Work Act.

An accident report form should contain the following information:

* details of the injured person (age, sex, occupation and contact details)
* date and time of the accident
* place where the accident occurred
* a brief description of the accident
* the nature of the injury
* the action taken
* signatures of all parties concerned (preferable).

The regulations under this legislation also require that if anyone is seriously injured or dies in connection with an accident in the workplace, or if anyone is off work for more than three days as a result of an accident at work, or if a specified occupational disease is certified by a doctor, then the employer must send a report to the Local Authority Environmental Health Department within seven days.

Employers Liability Act 1969

This legislation requires the employer to provide insurance cover against claims for injury or illness as a result of negligence by the employer or other employees.

A certificate of Employers Liability insurance must be displayed in the workplace.

Local Authority Bye-Laws

Local authorities may have their own legislation and local laws in relation to clinics providing services such as baby massage instruction.

However, the position is not uniform and will vary from County to County. It is therefore wise to seek the advice of the Local Authority Environmental Health Officer.

It is worth remembering that the Trading Standards and Environmental Health Departments at the Local Authority office will have a variety of leaflets and resources relating to legislation and these may be updated from time to time.

Consumer Legislation

It is important for instructors to be aware of the implications of consumer legislation, which is designed to protect any person who buys goods or services to ensure that:

* the goods are of merchantable quality
* the goods are not faulty
* there is an accurate description of the good or service.

The Sale of Goods Act 1979/The Supply of Goods and Services Act 1982

As consumers of products and services, clients have rights under the Sale of Goods Act 1979 and the Supply of Goods and Services Act 1982.

This legislation identifies the contract of sale, which takes place between the retailer (the clinic/salon) and the consumer (the client).

The Sale of Goods Act 1979 was the first of the laws and covers rights including the goods being accurately described without misleading the consumer.

The Supply of Goods and Services Act 1982 covers rights relating to the standards of service, in that goods and services provided should be of reasonable merchantable quality, described accurately, and be fit for their intended purpose.

The Act also requires that the service provided to a consumer should be carried out with reasonable skill and care, within a reasonable time and for a reasonable cost.

The Sale and Supply of Goods Act 1994

This legislation amends the previous Acts and has introduced guidelines on defining the quality of goods.

Consumer Protection Act 1987

This Act provides the consumer with protection when buying goods or services to ensure that products are safe for use on the client during the treatment, or are safe to be sold as a retail product.

The Act provides the same rights to anyone injured by a defective product, whether the product was sold to them or not.

The Act also covers giving misleading price indications about goods, services or facilities. The term price indication also includes price comparisons. To be misleading includes any wrongful indications about conditions attached to a price, about what you expect to happen to a price in the future and what you say in price comparisons.

It is essential to understand the implications of this legislation, including the promotion of special offers as it could result in legal proceedings.

Trade Descriptions Act 1968 (amended 1987)

This Act prohibits the use of false descriptions, or selling or offering the sale of goods that have been described falsely. This Act covers advertisements such as oral descriptions, display cards and applies to quality and quantity as well as fitness for purpose and price.

It is important to understand its provision, where the description is given by another person and repeated. Thus to repeat a manufacturer's claim is to be equally liable.

Data Protection Act 1984

This legislation protects clients' personal information being stored on a computer.

If client records are stored on computer, the establishment must be registered under this Act.

The Data Protection Act operates to ensure that the information stored is used only for the purposes for which it was given.

Businesses should therefore ensure that they:

* only hold information which is relevant
* allow individuals access to the information held on them
* prevent unauthorised access to the information.

Performing Rights Act

If the instructor is using relaxation music whilst carrying out baby massage instruction in a public place, it may be necessary to obtain a licence from Phonographic Performance Ltd (PPL) or the Performing Rights Society (PRS) which is a organisation that collects licence payments as royalties on behalf of performers and record companies, whose music is protected under the Copyright Designs and Patent Act 1998.

When seeking to play music in treatment premises it is important to check whether the music is 'copyright frcc', in which case no licence fee is due, or whether it is protected under this legislation.

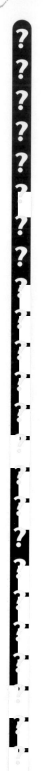

Questions for **R**eview

1. State four reasons why it is important to carry out a consultation with a parent/carer before instructing baby massage techniques

    _____
    _____
    _____
    _____

2. List five conditions that are contra-indicated to baby massage, stating the reason(s) why in each case

    _____
    _____
    _____
    _____
    _____
    _____
    _____
    _____

3. State three conditions that may require a GP's advice before proceeding with baby massage

    _____
    _____
    _____
    _____
    _____
    _____

4.   State how the following may affect the provision of baby massage

   i) recent immunisation

   _____

   _____

   ii) skin allergies

   _____

   _____

   iii) an unhealed navel

   _____

   _____

5.   List four caution sites that parents should be advised to avoid whilst massaging their baby

   _____

   _____

6.   State six points from the Code of Ethics for baby massage instructors

   _____

   _____

   _____

   _____

   _____

7.   Name two important pieces of legislation relevant to a baby massage instructor

   _____

   _____

   _____

   _____

07 *Baby Communication*

Baby Communication

The ability to communicate is one of the most important skills that a child acquires, as once developed it forms the basis for subsequent learning and is the medium through which relationships are formed in life.

Long before a baby can say their first words, communication takes places between infants and their parents. Communicating with a baby involves touching, holding, rocking, talking, active listening and learning to synchronise with the baby's behaviour.

This chapter explores the different ways baby states may be interpreted by instructors and parents. Baby massage is in itself a unique form of communication and through correctly identifying a baby's state responses may be adapted to enhance bonding and attachment.

This chapter explores the different ways in which babies communicate their needs.

At the end of this chapter you will be able to relate the following knowledge to your role as instructor/parent/carer:

❋ The different types of infant states

❋ The language of crying and identifying a baby's cry

❋ Interpreting and responding to a baby's cues.

Infant States

A baby's response to massage will be very much influenced by their behavioural state at the time at which the session is introduced.

The different forms of infant states may be identified as:

❋ deep sleep

❋ light sleep

❋ drowsy

❋ quiet alert

❋ active alert

❋ crying.

Deep Sleep State

In a deep sleep state, there will be little or no movement, although the baby may twitch periodically. The eyes will not move and breathing will be regular.

As there will be little or no feedback in this state, it is not recommended to give massage when a baby is in the deep sleep state.

Light Sleep State

In this state, there will be some movement from the baby; eyelids may flutter and there will be rapid eye movement. The baby may fuss briefly and may suck or smile.

Breathing will be irregular.

As there will be minimal response, little or no feedback, it is not recommended to commence massage when a baby is in a light sleep state.

Drowsy State

In this state, a baby may exhibit a varied activity level; movements will be generally smooth with mild startles. Eyes may be open and closed and will appear heavy and glazed. Breathing will be irregular and responses will be delayed.

In this state, a massage may be approached in two possible ways: brisker strokes to arouse the baby to a quiet alert state or slower to help induce sleep.

Quiet Alert State

In a quiet alert state, a baby may show either a little or a lot of movement.

This is the most attentive and focused state as the eyes will appear open, wide and bright. Breathing will be regular and the baby's face will appear bright and shiny.

This is the ideal time for interaction with baby massage.

Active Alert State

In this state there will be much movement and the baby may fuss. Eyes will appear open but less bright than in a quiet alert state. Breathing will be irregular and there will be an increased sensitivity to internal and external stimuli.

In this state, a baby may tolerate slow massage strokes to help calm and lower their state or they may benefit from a more active routine which includes rhythm and movement.

Massage may need to be modified or stopped according to the infant's response and tolerance levels.

Crying

Crying is an important and effective means of communication for a baby and is a powerful way of alerting a carer to their needs. When crying, babies tend to exhibit more body movement and may change colour (often becoming red in the face). Eyes may be tightly closed or open. The baby tends to grimace and there will be increased irregularity of breathing.

Massage should not be commenced whilst a baby is crying. If a baby cries throughout the session, the massage must be stopped to comfort/feed/adjust the positioning of the baby, and may be recommended if the baby is responsive.

Identifying a Baby's Cries

It can be a challenging task to parents to determine which cries require attention from them and when a baby may be left to self-calm.

There are various types of cries that are usually distinct enough to be categorised:

Hunger

A demanding, incessant, urgent cry. This is usually a typically short, rhythmical and explosive cry. If unattended, a hunger cry may develop into an anger or intense pain cry.

Anger

This type of cry has a sustained, low pitch and has a vibrato quality to it. The baby's lips may appear tightly clenched with the open mouth cry, as if in pain. There may also be a snarled expression and an arching of the back.

Tiredness

This type of cry may be interpreted as non-urgent and less rhythmical than a hunger cry. This type of cry is often described as 'fussing' and will tend to occur when a baby is overloaded with too much stimuli, or is simply tired.

The baby will often attempt to console themselves by touching their ears, touching their hair or sucking their fingers. They may also rub their eyes. They will not wish to engage in any activity and may turn away from their parent/carer.

Pain or Discomfort

This is a piercing, sharp, penetrating cry (may be a sharp anguished scream followed by a brief period of apnea (no breathing)), which usually continues even after a baby is picked up. This type of cry has a sharp intense shrill to it and is designed to demand an immediate response from the parent/carer.

Boredom

A whiny, low-pitched hollow cry. It may be accompanied by the occasional pause as the baby anticipates the parent/carer attending to them. This cry is usually a signal that a baby needs a change of position, or activity or a different type of interaction.

Most babies develop what is often referred to as a 'fussy period' towards the end of the day. This can be interpreted as adaptive behaviour, and is an essential part of a baby's daily reorganisation of their nervous system.

Babies have immature nervous systems that can take in and utilise stimuli throughout the day, but there will always be a tendency towards overload. As the day proceeds, an increasingly overloaded nervous system begins to cycle in shorter and shorter sleep and feeding periods. After this is over, the nervous system needs to 'let off steam' in order to reorganise itself.

After the fussy period is over, the baby will seem better organised in sleeping and eating in more regular rhythms. During this frustrating 'fussy period' it can be tempting for parents to overhandle their babies and get anxious and frantic over what appears to be excessive crying.

Babies need to learn to be able to handle their own stresses, and carers getting anxious about fussing and crying tends to increase the amount and intensity of it!

Cutting down on excess stimuli and avoiding overhandling is often the best solution to allow the baby to establish its own pattern for self-calming and self-comforting.

Responding to a baby's cues

Observing a baby's non-verbal communication and interpreting their cues are just as important as verbal communication. A baby's non-verbal signs may be shown in:

* their body posture
* gestures and body movements
* facial expressions

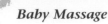

* eye contact

* tone of their cry or verbal expression.

Learning to respond to a baby's cues is essential to parents interpreting their readiness for baby massage.

Babies use two main types of verbal and non-verbal communication to indicate their readiness for interaction:

* engagement

* disengagement.

Engagement

Signs of readiness for interaction may be in the form of subtle or strong signals. It is important for parents to look for the verbal and non-verbal cues before commencing the massage.

Subtle signs of engagement include:

* facial expressions—eyes may widen, eyebrows may raise and the face may brighten

* head and eye movements—the baby's head may lift and their eyes may turn towards their parent/carer

* hand and finger movements—hands may be open with fingers relaxed and slightly flexed.

Strong signs of engagement include:

* smiling

* sustained eye contact with the parent/carer

* verbal cues—babbling, talking, feeding sounds.

Disengagement

Instructors and parents need to be aware of the subtle and strong signs of disengagement in order to respect the baby's wishes and modify the massage interaction.

Subtle signs of disengagement are usually a sign that a baby needs a break in the interaction and this should be respected before the signs become stronger.

Subtle signs of disengagement include:

* eyes turning away from the parent/carer

* facial grimacing

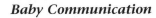

✳ whimpering or yawning

✳ lowering of the head and eyes closing

✳ raising of the shoulders

✳ increased body movements

✳ limbs straightening tightly.

Strong signs of disengagement include:

✳ crying or fussing

✳ turning the head away

✳ arching of the back

✳ pushing a parent/carer's hands away

✳ pulling away, rolling, crawling or walking away!

Interpreting the above cues will help the instructor and parent to determine the baby's readiness for massage and the baby's responsiveness throughout the massage.

This will help a parent to become more responsive to their baby's needs, as by actively responding to the baby's cues the massage interaction will become a more positive experience for both parent and baby.

Questions for Review

1. State three ways in which parents communicate with their babies through massage

_____

_____

_____

2. State three ways in which a baby's non-verbal signs may be shown

_____

_____

_____

3. Why is it important for parents to interpret and respond to their baby's non-verbal, as well as verbal cues, throughout a massage session?

_____

_____

_____

_____

_____

_____

4. Which is the ideal infant state in which to commence massage interaction?

_____

_____

_____

5. Outline how the following baby cries may be interpreted:

i) hunger

_____

_____

_____

ii) tiredness/overstimulation

_____

_____

_____

iii) pain or discomfort

_____

_____

_____

6.   i) State three signs of engagement that could indicate a baby's readiness for massage

_____

_____

_____

ii) State three signs of disengagement that would indicate it was an inappropriate time to commence or continue massage

_____

_____

_____

08 *Preparing for Baby Massage*

Preparing for Baby Massage

When preparing for baby massage, it is important to create the right atmosphere in order that it is a pleasant and rewarding experience for both parent and baby.

It is also essential that the parent/carer feels relaxed and comfortable before massaging their baby, in order to make it an enjoyable experience.

An instructor's role involves advising parents/carers on how to prepare the environment for massage and how they may prepare themselves in order to ensure a continuity of the schedule at home.

At the end of this chapter you will be able to relate the following knowledge to your role as an instructor/parent/carer:

❋ Preparing the ideal environment for baby massage

❋ Advantages and disadvantages of different massage supports

❋ Parental positioning for baby massage

❋ Hygiene precautions

❋ Safety precautions and avoiding hazards

❋ Suitable mediums for baby massage

❋ Relaxation techniques for parents

Preparing the Ideal Environment for Baby Massage

Where to Massage

When advising a parent on preparing for baby massage, suggest they pick an area of the home where they enjoy spending time together.

The temperature of the room is a primary consideration and needs to be roughly 10°C above normal (babies lose their body heat ten times more quickly than adults).

The following advice should be given to a parent/carer as a preparation checklist before massaging.

✻ Clear a comfortable space to work in, which is free from obstructions, wires and unprotected plugs

✻ Ensure that the room is warm and that doors are closed to reduce draughts

✻ Avoid lights that are too bright and glaring

✻ Clear pets from the room

✻ Play some soft music to create a relaxing atmosphere

✻ Ensure that you will remain undisturbed for the duration of the massage session

✻ Allow plenty of time, so you do not feel rushed or stressed.

Resource Checklist for Baby Massage

✻ Several soft pillows/cushions to use as supports for your back and supports for your baby.

✻ Plenty of medium to large soft towels at hand to keep the baby warm, as baby's temperature will drop during the massage. Keep a warm blanket (preferably made from soft cotton) to wrap the baby up in after the massage.

✻ Dry hand cleanser to cleanse hands before and after the massage.

✻ Oil/lotion in a small leakproof container.

✻ Tissues or kitchen roll in order to remove any excess oil/lotion from your hands.

✻ Supply of nappies and baby wipes (the relaxation of the massage often makes a baby empty their bladder).

✻ A few soft toys near by to stimulate your baby if he or she becomes distracted throughout the massage.

✻ Have a bottle prepared for your baby for after the massage (cooled boiled water is recommended) although it is perfectly natural to breast feed or bottle feed after a massage.

Parental Positioning for Baby Massage

It is essential that parents/carers are comfortable before commencing massage with their babies. Instructors will need to discuss different positions that allow parents to keep their backs straight and avoid discomfort throughout the massage.

It is also worth considering that parental positioning and baby position will inevitably change as the baby develops, and adaptability will be needed.

Different Massage Supports for Baby Massage

There is a variety of supports for parents to try, the advantages and disadvantages of both are discussed below:

Bed

Advantages

* May be a more comfortable environment for baby and parent to relax in (conducive to relaxation).
* May be more spacious.
* More supportive (head boards, pillows, soft surface).
* Suitable when combined with a bedtime routine.

Disadvantages

* Safety—baby may roll off.

Floor

Advantages

* Easily accessible support (parents spend a great deal of their time on the floor with their babies).
* Plenty of space (will depend on environment).

Disadvantages

* May be uncomfortable for parent/carer.

When using the floor or bed as a support for baby massage the following positions may be tried by parents to see which is comfortable for them:

Sitting with Legs Straddled

Use a hard surface such as a wall or a sofa as a back support and secure a large cushion behind the back. Sit with the legs stretched out on either side of the baby.

Sitting with legs straddled ▼

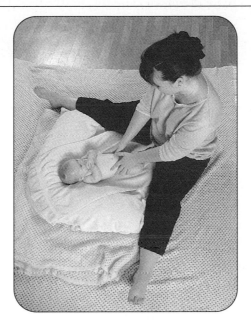

Kneeling

Use a pillow or soft towel under your knees and one under your bottom and sit back into a comfortable position.

Kneeling ▼

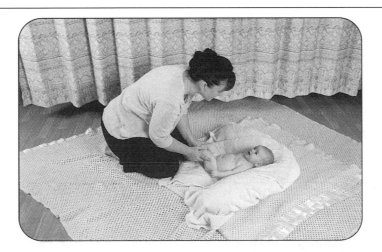

Legs Crossed

Sit on a soft cushion or pillow with your legs crossed.

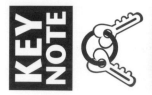

With the above positions it may also be preferable to elevate the position of the baby by securing pillows behind, and underneath, in order that you can maintain eye contact and avoid leaning over too much.

Lap

Advantages

❋ Good position for very young or small babies (they may feel more secure).

Disadvantages

❋ Not such a comfortable position for older babies (may roll off).

❋ May be uncomfortable or restrictive for the parent.

Plinth

Advantages

❋ May be a more comfortable working height (parent sits on chair opposite plinth).

❋ Height can be adjusted by parent/instructor.

❋ Could be more comfortable for parent/carer with a disability or a mother who has had a Caesarean.

Disadvantages

❋ Safety—baby may fall off.

❋ Cost implications.

❋ Not readily accessible.

❋ Doesn't allow as much 'closeness'.

❋ Unsuitable support if baby is large.

❋ Plinth takes up space.

Hygiene and Safety Precautions

Parents/carers and instructors should observe the following hygiene and safety precautions prior to the massage session.

Hygiene Precautions for Baby Massage

❋ Always wash hands before and after commencing the massage (dry hand cleansers are ideal).

❋ Ensure that all jewellery that may scratch baby has been removed.

❋ Wear comfortable loose clothing and tie hair back during the massage.

❋ Make sure that nails are short and won't scratch the delicate skin of the baby. Also remove varnish from nails which may react with the baby's skin.

❋ Check that the baby has no infectious conditions that may be spread by the massage.

Safety Precautions for Baby Massage

❋ Always refer to a qualified instructor if unsure about whether to, or how to massage the baby. Refer to the baby's GP if the baby has a medical condition.

❋ Avoid massaging the baby if you are suffering from a cold, flu or infectious illness.

❋ Prepare a safe environment for the massage session—avoid massaging in front of open fires or on a slippery surface.

❋ Avoid having hot drinks in the area.

❋ Keep oil away from baby's face.

❋ Keep massage oil in a small leakproof bottle.

❋ If using oil to massage the baby, ensure all residue is removed before lifting him/her up by wrapping baby up in a soft towel.

When to Massage

Babies love repetition and like to anticipate what comes next. It is therefore best to be consistent in timing, setting, and the time of day.

It is best for parents to allow plenty of time so that they do not feel hurried or stressed before starting the massage.

Baby massage can be carried out at any time of the day, although it is best to advise parents to massage between feeds to avoid discomfort due to their baby being too full or hungry during the massage. The massage may be incorporated into part of a nightime/winding down bathtime routine, or may be integrated into daily schedules such as changing, washing or story time.

Depending on their family circumstances, parents can be encouraged to fit the massage in when they have time to enjoy it with their baby, without having to consider other family duties.

Parental Relaxation Techniques

Babies have the ability, even from a very early age, to detect tension and anxiety in their parents and then absorb it. It is, therefore, worth parents taking time out to relax themselves before starting the massage session with their baby. If parents can learn to release their own tensions, the baby will tend to respond more positively to touch.

If both baby and parent are happy and relaxed when commencing the massage, they will associate this feeling with massage and it will, therefore, help to make it a positive experience they will both want to repeat time and time again.

Relaxation Exercises for Parents

Below are two breathing exercises which may be taught to parents to help them relax and focus before starting to massage their baby.

Learning to breathe properly enables the body to relax and regain its natural balance, whilst calming the mind and reducing tension and anxiety.

Breathing Exercise 1

Sit in a comfortable position and loosen tight clothing.

Place one hand on the chest and the other across the stomach.

Inhale deeply through the nose to fill the upper chest cavity and down to the lower part of the lungs, as if breathing into the stomach for a count of 6.

Exhale slowly to a count of 12, allowing the air to escape from the top of your lungs first before the lower part deflates.

Repeat this exercise 6–8 times.

Breathing Exercise 2

Apply the first two fingers of the right hand to the side of the right nostril and press gently to close it. Breathe in slowly through the left nostril and hold for a count of 3.

Transfer the first two fingers to the left nostril to close it.

Calendula

This is especially suitable for use on babies with very sensitive skins as it has anti-inflammatory, softening, soothing and healing properties. It is suitable for all skin types, but especially for dry and sensitive.

Coconut Oil

This is a popular oil for baby massage in Indian cultures. It is perfect for baby massage as it is a light oil, which is very moisturising and softening on the skin.

Grapeseed Oil

This oil is suitable for all skin types and is a gentle emollient, which can help babies' skin to retain moisture. Contains linoleic acid, protein and a small proportion of vitamin E; it is free from cholesterol. Grapeseed oil is an effective medium for baby massage as it is light and penetrates the skin quickly.

Jojoba

This oil has a light and fine texture and is therefore suitable for baby massage. It has anti-inflammatory properties and is suitable for sensitive skins.

It is highly penetrative, rich in vitamin E, protein and minerals and is a natural moisturiser for babies' skin.

Olive Oil

This oil is suitable for dry, dehydrated or inflamed skins. It contains a good source of vitamin E and is very soothing for baby massage.

Sunflower Oil

This oil is suitable for all skin types, especially dry. It is excellent for baby massage as it is a light oil and contains high levels of vitamin E.

Preblended Baby Massage Oils

There are a number of companies that sell massage oils for babies and children that have been preblended with essential oils in a base oil such as sweet almond, jojoba or sunflower.

It is recommended that these oils are not used until a baby is at least 3-months-old and that if a child's skin is very sensitive, a patch test is carried out before using the oil. Essential oils can be beneficial in helping with typical babyhood problems, however due to their concentrated nature it is advisable that parents use preblended oils only if they are being advised by a qualified aromatherapist. See Resource Section for a suitable list of suppliers.

Massage Gels

Massage gels are an alternative to massaging with oil and will provide an equal amount of slip for massage, as they are oil based. When using gel, only a small amount will be required to give the desired effect.

It is also important to ensure that any residue has been removed after the massage as it will tend to be more slippery in nature.

Massage Creams

If a baby's skin is dry then it may be advisable for parents to massage with a cream, preferably one that is light and easily absorbed, with a high proportion of vitamin E.

If parents are used to applying a certain cream to treat their baby's skin condition, then using the cream as a massage medium would be a useful way of combining the daily routine.

Massage Lotions

Lotions tend to have a higher proportion of water and therefore, depending on ingredients and consistency, may be suitable as a massage medium.

Avent sell a lotion which is marketed as a baby cleanser/moisturiser, and is an effective massage medium (contains avocado oil, shea butter and milk proteins).

Questions for **R**eview

1. List four considerations when preparing the environment for baby massage

    _____

    _____

    _____

    _____

    _____

2. List four hygiene precautions to consider when carrying out baby massage

    _____

    _____

    _____

    _____

    _____

3. List six safety precautions when carrying out baby massage

    _____

    _____

    _____

    _____

    _____

4. State the benefits of using the following mediums with baby massage

    i) Coconut oil

    _____

    _____

    ii) Almond oil

    _____

    _____

iii) Sunflower oil

_____

_____

5. Discuss the advantages and disadvantages of using the following massage supports for baby massage

i) Lap

_____

_____

_____

_____

_____

_____

ii) Bed

_____

_____

_____

_____

_____

iii) Plinth

_____

_____

_____

_____

_____

Baby Massage Techniques 09

Baby Massage Techniques

Touch is an important part of a baby's physical and emotional growth and is said to be as important to babies as food in their need for survival.

Learning baby massage is an ideal way of encouraging parents to extend their natural inclination to cuddle and caress their babies. It is one of the most valuable skills a parent can learn as it is an immediate, convenient, and preventative resource that, above all, costs very little to perform.

It is also one of the most long-lasting skills a parent can adopt as it may be used to benefit a child from birth through to adulthood.

This chapter outlines the practical skills to help parents/carers to massage their babies. Although the techniques are illustrated in a set routine parents may be encouraged to use them as a guideline and to develop their own style of massage to suit their baby's needs.

At the end of this chapter you will be able to relate the following knowledge to your role as instructor/parent/carer:

* The different types of massage techniques used in baby massage and how they differ in terms of pressure and application
* Positioning techniques for baby massage
* The use of music and movement to complement baby massage sessions
* Practical baby massage techniques
* Guidelines and adaptations for babies of different ages—0–3 months, 3–6 months, 6–9 months, 9–12 months , 12–15 months, 15–18 months and beyond
* The importance of stretching techniques and mobility exercises with baby massage
* The challenge of massaging twins
* Common baby ailments and how baby massage can help

* Common reactions and outcomes to baby massage
* Evaluate feedback from babies and parents
* Frequency and timing
* After care advice.

Massage Movements used in Baby Massage

Effleurage/Stroking

This is one of the main techniques used in baby massage.

The effleurage stroke is a smooth, gliding and flowing stroke that follows the contours of a baby's body. Both hands may work simultaneously on larger body parts and one hand, thumbs or fingers may work best on smaller areas.

It is a long gliding stroke that enables the parent/carer to introduce their hands to the baby and apply the massage medium, if applicable. It is generally a lightly performed stroke that maintains the continuity of the massage routine by indicating to the baby which parts of the body are about to be massaged.

It soothes, relaxes and lightly increases the circulation and is used as a linking stroke in between other movements.

When using this technique on a very young baby, it is often the fingers that maintain the contact, rather than the whole palmar surface due to the surface area of the baby.

A light touch is all that should be applied initially and a medium to firmer pressure may be applied once the baby has increased in size and has become accustomed to the feeling of touch massage.

Petrissage/Kneading

This technique involves kneading a baby's tissues by lifting, rolling and squeezing them with the fingers and thumbs.

The application of petrissage is more focused and less generalised than effleurage, and is performed on the more fleshy areas of a baby's body.

Depending on the area being massaged, petrissage may be applied with one hand or by using both hands alternately. For smaller areas, kneading may be achieved by using the fingers and thumbs. Pressure should be smoothly and firmly applied and then relaxed; hands then glide onto an adjacent area and the movement is repeated.

This technique will help to release tension in a baby's muscles, and will help to increase the absorption of nutrients into the tissue and the elimination of waste from the tissues.

NB. It is important that a baby has sufficient tissue density before this technique is applied.

Frictions

These are circular movements applied with the pad of the thumbs or fingers over a small area of the baby's skin. Light pressure is applied on a baby, in contrast to the application of massage in an adult.

Frictions will help to release tension, increase the circulation locally to the area and aid elimination of waste.

Gentle stretching and joint movement

Gentle stretching and joint movements may be used after a baby's muscles have relaxed sufficiently and are performed towards the end of the massage session; although they may be interspersed throughout the massage provided the limbs and joints to be stretched are relaxed.

The use of gentle stretching and joint movement will help to increase joint mobility, maintain flexibility of joints, as well as increase the development of muscular strength and suppleness.

They are also a useful tool to use to punctuate the massage routine to add variety and fun, particularly as the baby develops and becomes more aware of their body movements.

NB. It is important when carrying out gentle stretching or gentle joint movement that you have the baby's full co-operation and that they are relaxed, otherwise the baby may experience discomfort and disengage from the interaction.

Positioning Techniques for Baby Massage

Positioning during baby massage will depend on the baby's age, physical development, and above all their comfort and preference (as well as the comfort of the parent). The most common position for baby massage is when a baby is lying face-up (supine) or face-down (prone).

Baby Facing Up

This is an ideal position for baby massage as it provides the best opportunity for interaction and eye contact during the massage. The baby can be supported by a soft cushion, pillow or mat.

Baby Facing Down

This is the preferred position when massaging the back, although most babies do not like being placed on their stomachs (this is mainly due to the fact that it is stressed to parents to ensure their baby sleeps on either their back or their side and babies therefore are not so used to lying on their front).

In this position the baby may be supported as when facing-up, with a soft cushion, pillow or mat. Alternatively babies may be placed over the parent's/carer's lap.

Baby Side Lying

This position is when parents are lying on a bed or on the floor and cuddling in with their baby. In this position the back, abdomen and legs may be massaged comfortably for both parent and baby. As both are lying down, it is the most preferable position when massage is encouraged to induce relaxation and sleep.

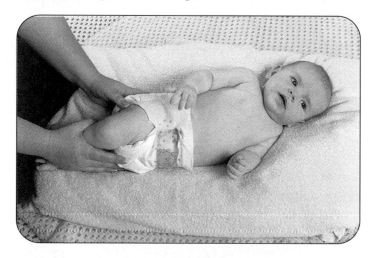

Baby Sitting

This position is useful for an older and more mobile baby. Sitting affords more freedom to play and the session can become highly interactive by introducing play games with the hands throughout the massage.

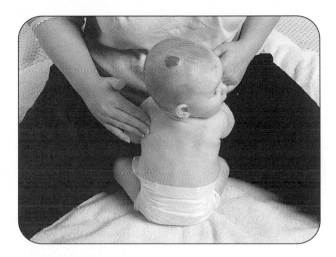

Baby Over the Shoulder

This is an ideal position for very tiny babies or those who need to be comforted and held, as there is closer contact with their parent's/carer's body.

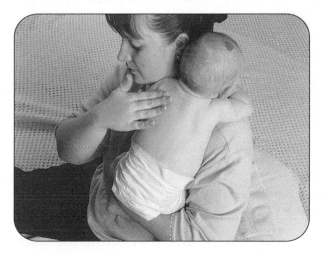

The Use of Music and Movement to Complement Baby Massage Sessions

Music can be a great source of stress relief to babies and their parents and is a valuable accompaniment to massage.

There are CDs that have been especially composed to soothe and calm young babies and children. The type of music best suited to massage is one which has a repetitive element that babies can quickly relate to and over time it will become a comforting sound that they associate with the warmth of the massage and being close to their parent/carer. See Resource section at the end of the book for suitable titles for baby massage.

The Use of Movement and Music with Massage

Singing songs with massage is a fun way to extend the massage experience with babies. Babies also find the sound of their parent's voice singing very comforting and reassuring, as well as enjoyable, as it is another opportunity for interaction and increased vocalisation.

For an older baby, the music of song and movement can help to add variety and can at the same time help their physical and language development.

Singing songs or nursery rhymes is a very enjoyable and unthreatening way to help children to develop speech using appropriate words and speech patterns. When children learn a nursery rhyme they have to actively listen to it, memorise it, and repeat it back. All these skills collectively help to develop a child's language and are a progression to developing linguistic structures for thinking.

Nursery rhymes are rich in language and repetition. The repetition of vowel sounds, consonants and made-up words helps a young child's ability to speak.

Babies and young children love repetition and like to repeat the same sound over and over again; this gives them the opportunity to play and practise with language skills.

The combination of singing and movement in time to the music provides babies and young children with an opportunity to develop and practise their fine and gross motor skills and increase their understanding of how their bodies work.

The music or song can be reinforced in conjunction with the direction of the massage movement or stretch (i.e. when carrying out the gentle joint movement of the hips in a circular direction this can be done to singing 'The wheels on the bus go round and round'). The movement encompassing the whole of the body like the connecting stroke can be combined with 'Head, and shoulders, knees and toes . . .' helping the child to relate to parts of their body.

All nursery rhymes are patterns of rhythms that are based on counting. When young children learn nursery rhymes they have to remember all the patterns. This is a stepping stone to a future understanding of maths. Lots of nursery rhymes have actions to do with directions (up, down etc), and this helps children to understand and learn mathematical concepts.

The massage movements can be used in the same way by parents counting the strokes as well as reinforcing the parts being massaged.

Pointers for Parents/Carers Before Massaging

❋ Ensure that all resources are to hand (oil, blanket, towels, baby's drink/bottle/comforter/soft toy).

❋ Ensure that you and your baby are in a comfortable position.

❋ Ensure that you feel relaxed (if necessary carry out some relaxation techniques before starting).

❋ Maintain contact with your baby at all times during the massage to ensure continuity.

❋ Smile and talk softly to your baby throughout the massage, explain and reassure him or her of what you are about to do.

❋ The intonation of voice is very important throughout the massage and will help your baby to interpret the experiences.

❋ Observe and respond to your baby's cues throughout the massage.

❋ Try to use a slow rhythmical pace, which will be relaxing for both you and your baby.

❋ Use a light and soft pressure to start with and be guided by your instinct and your baby regarding increasing the pressure.

❋ If your baby becomes distressed throughout the massage, stop and try again later.

❋ Try to relax and remember that the experience belongs to you and your baby and should be enjoyable for the parent and the baby.

❋ Crying helps babies to communicate how they are feeling, and can be a form of healthy release in that the baby may be releasing pent-up anguish.

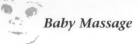

Baby Massage Techniques

5-Minute Baby Massage Routine

Note for Instructors

For parents with little or no experience of massage, it is important to start to introduce their babies to massage gradually. It is recommended that a first massage experience is relatively short in duration to assess the baby's reactions and tolerance, and the parents' attention span.

Note for Parents

The objective of the following routine is to help familiarise yourself and your baby with gentle touch and massage. Once you are familiar with the techniques it will generally only take about 5–10 minutes at home.

* Ensure that you have everything you need to hand before starting.
* Wipe your hands with a dry hand cleanser/wipes.
* Start by getting the baby's attention and talking softly and gently.
* Relax your hands and fingers.
* When massaging an area of your baby's body with one hand, use the other hand to support and reassure your baby.

Apply a small amount of oil to the palm of the hand and rub together to warm.

It is important to ask your baby's permission before commencing the massage, as this demonstrates a sense of respect and teaches the baby to set his or her own touch boundaries that are comfortable and controlled.

Massage Techniques to the Front of Baby's Body

Start by preparing a safe and comfortable work surface. If working on the floor, it is important to work against a hard surface and be supported by pillows to ensure comfort. See pages 142–4 for details of comfortable positioning.

Lay a protective sheet on the floor/table/couch/bed and on top of this maybe a soft support such as a changing mat or pillow/cushions covered by two towels (one large and one medium sized). Positioning may initially present a challenge and this may vary from baby to baby, and will change as the massage progresses and the baby grows.

When you are ready slowly remove your baby's clothing and nappy in preparation for commencing.

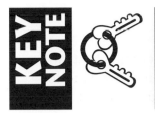

If your baby feels uncomfortable having his or her clothes removed initially for massage, the techniques described below may also be carried out through soft clothing such as a sleepsuit; some of the techniques may even be adapted for use in the massage with the help of a wash/bath mitt.

Lay your baby on his or her back to start the massage.

Connecting Stroke to the Front of Baby's Body

1   With both hands start with a long sweeping effleurage stroke gently across the top of baby's chest and shoulders, down the arms, lightly back up the arms and then stroke down the trunk to the legs and feet. Without breaking contact reverse the stroke from the feet up, the legs, across the trunk and chest and down the arms with a feather-like touch. Repeat × 6.

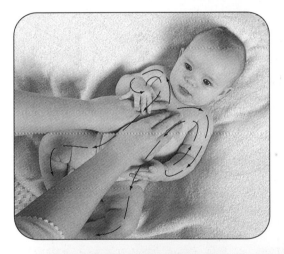

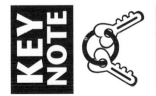

The connecting stroke helps parents to establish contact and connect with their babies' bodies before commencing the massage

Baby's Chest

X Stroke to the Front of the Chest

2 Using one hand stroke from the top of your baby's shoulder and chest, and gently lift as you stroke across to the opposite hip (use your other hand to support the baby at the hip). Without breaking contact repeat this on the other side (as if drawing an X stroke across the front of baby's body). Repeat × 6.

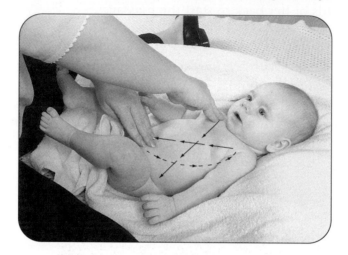

Little Circles to Baby's Chest

3 Perform light circles with the pads of the fingers of both hands across the top of the baby's chest muscles, starting from the inside and progressing outwards to the top of the arms. Repeat × 3.

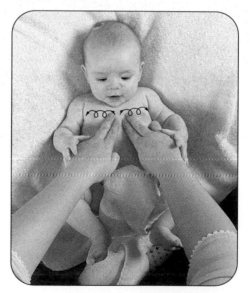

Butterfly Strokes to the Chest

4 Use the weight of your relaxed hands across baby's chest, stroke both hands from the centre of chest outwards (as if drawing butterflies wings). Repeat the same stroke slightly further down, slightly overlapping the previous stroke. Repeat × 3.

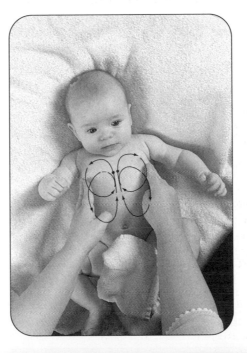

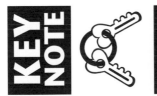

KEY NOTE

Massaging your baby's chest helps to relax the chest muscles and aid your baby's breathing. It can also help to clear congestion.

Baby's Arms

Glide and Stretch to Arms

5 Taking one arm at a time, using alternate hands (one to support your baby's hands and lift the arm slightly away from the body, and one to massage) gently stroke from the baby's hands up the arm and circle around the top of arm, returning back down with a lighter stroke, gently stretching as you glide down. Repeat × 3.

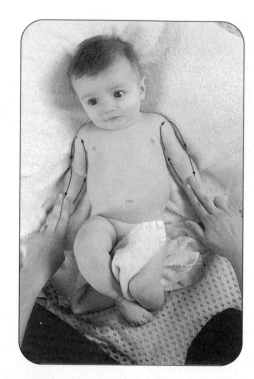

Little Circles to Baby's Palms

6 Taking one hand at a time, perform little circles with the thumbs into the baby's palm, gently stretching the hands open as you massage. Repeat × 3.

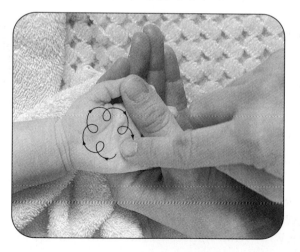

Gentle Squeeze to the Fingers

7 Taking one finger at a time between the thumb and forefinger gently massage and gently squeeze and release. Repeat × 1.

Squeeze and Release to Both Arms

8   When both arms have been massaged gently squeeze and release the arm muscles working from the top of the arms down to the hands. Repeat × 3.

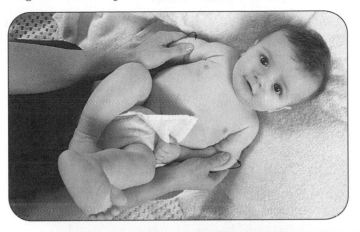

KEY NOTE

A baby's posture from birth means that their arms tend to be flexed and closed in towards their body.

Massaging your baby's arms can help to open out the chest and shoulder and increase flexibility, suppleness and co-ordination in their limbs.

Baby's Abdomen

Circles around Baby's Navel

9   Using the weight of your relaxed hand to rest gently on baby's abdomen, perform gentle circles around the navel with the pads of the fingers in a clockwise circular direction. Repeat × 3.

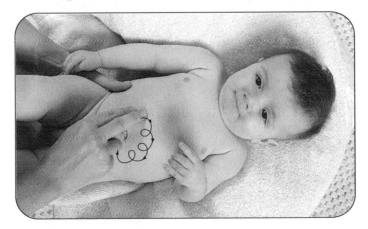

NB. Take care not to use excessive pressure here to avoid causing discomfort by pressing too hard over the baby's bladder and intestines.

Gentle Circular Stroking to the Solar Plexus

10 Using the weight of a relaxed hand, perform little circles in a clockwise direction under the bottom of the baby's rib cage (in the centre of the upper abdomen). Repeat × 3.

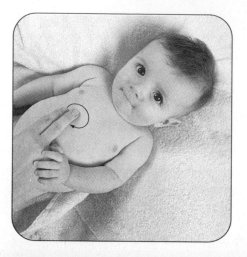

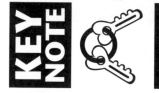

KEY NOTE

Massaging your baby's abdomen can help to ease colicky pains, ease constipation and digestion. It can also help to relieve your baby's anxiety as by massaging the abdomen it increases the volume of air inhaled into your baby's lungs.

Front of Baby's Legs

Glide and Stretch to Baby's Legs

11 Taking one leg at a time, using alternate hands, gently stroke from the baby's foot up the leg and circle around the hips, returning back down with a lighter stroke, gently stretching as you glide down (use one hand to massage your baby's leg and the other hand to support and slightly lift the leg). Repeat × 3.

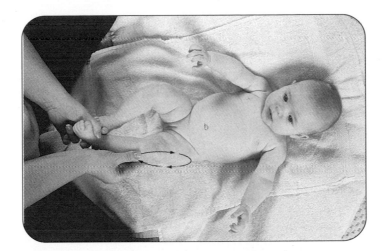

Little Circles into Sole of Baby's Foot

12 Taking one foot at a time, perform little circles with the thumbs into the sole of the baby's foot. Repeat × 3.

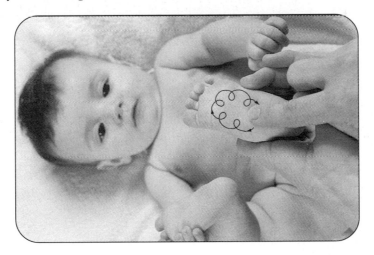

Gentle Squeeze of the Toes

13 Take one toe at a time and give a gentle massage between the thumb and fingers and then gently squeeze as you release them. Repeat × 1.

Squeeze and Release to Baby's Legs

14 Holding both legs, use the hands to gently squeeze and release the leg muscles working from the top of the thighs downwards. Repeat × 3.

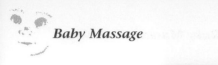

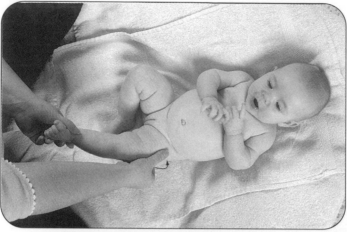

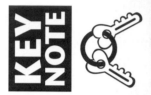 Massaging your baby's legs can help your baby to develop the strength and co-ordination for upright postures such as sitting, standing and walking. It will also help your baby to develop flexibility in his or her hip and knee joints.

Now turn your baby onto his or her front. The baby may either lie on the floor or other surface or may be placed across your lap.

Connecting Stroke to the Back of Baby's Body

15 With both hands perform a long sweeping effleurage stroke gently across the back of the baby's shoulders, down the back of the arms, brush back up the arms and then stroke down the back to the legs and feet. Without breaking contact reverse the stroke from the feet up the back of the legs, across the back and shoulders and down the arms with a feather-like touch. Repeat × 6.

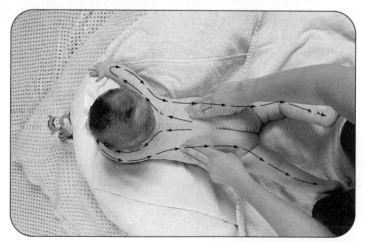

X-Stroke to the Back of Baby's Body

16 Stroke from top of the baby's shoulder and gently lift as you stroke across to the back of the opposite hip; without breaking contact repeat this the other side (as if drawing a X stroke across the back of baby's body). Repeat × 6.

Little Circles Either Side of Baby's Spine

17 Using the pads of the fingers of both hands, perform circular frictions either side of the spine. Repeat × 3.

NB. Take care to avoid pressure on the baby's spine.

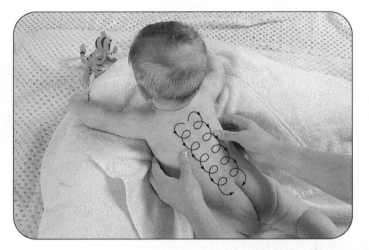

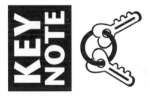

KEY NOTE

Massaging your baby's back will help your baby's spine to become strong and flexible. It will also help to stretch the front of the body as it will encourage deeper breathing and relax his or her abdomen.

Baby's Buttocks

Little Circles to the Buttocks

18 Perform little circles with both hands using the pads of the fingers, working from the centre of the buttock outwards towards the back of baby's hip. Repeat × 3.

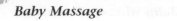
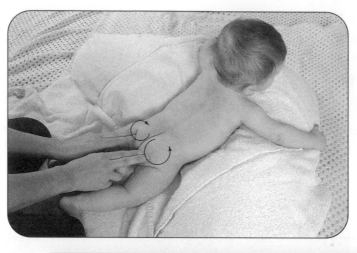

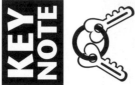 Massaging your baby's buttocks can help your baby to develop suppleness and flexibility in the lower back and hips for good posture.

Connecting Stroke to the Back of Baby's Body

19 Repeat the connecting stroke as in no: 15. Repeat × 6.

Now turn your baby back onto his or her back

Connecting Stroke to the Front of the Body

20 Repeat the connecting stroke as in no: 1 and stroke down the front of the body. Repeat × 6.

Bicycles

21 Finish with gentle stretching of legs (bicycle movements with the legs).

NB. Avoid this stretch if your baby has any hip problems.

At the end of the massage, advise the parent or carer to wrap their baby up in a towel, give them a kiss and a cuddle and a drink and when ready remove the oil before dressing.

Baby Stretches

It is important to ensure that stretches are only performed when your baby's muscles are warm and relaxed.

Stretching a baby's limbs helps them to develop flexibility by mobilising their joints. Babies usually enjoy the stretches and gentle joint movement when they are combined with playful noises or nursery rhymes.

Developing flexibility in the joints is very important to a baby's posture and for body suppleness. Certain stretches of the legs can help a baby with colic and constipation by releasing trapped wind.

The stretches illustrated below may be carried out throughout the massage routine or may be performed in a sequence at the end, depending on the baby's needs.

Arm Stretch

Holding baby's arms at the wrist, stretch them out to the sides and then cross the chest one way and then the other way.

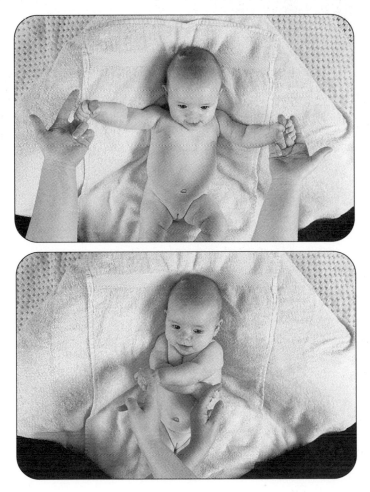

Arm and Leg Stretch

Hold one arm at the wrist and the opposite leg at the ankle. Bring them both into the centre and then release back out. Repeat on the other side.

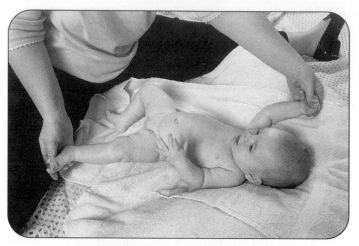

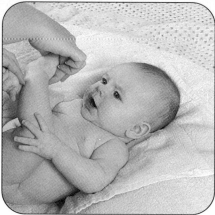

Leg Stretches (helpful for constipation, trapped wind, colic)

a) Hold the baby's legs at the ankles and cross them over as you bring them towards the abdomen. Then stretch them out straight.

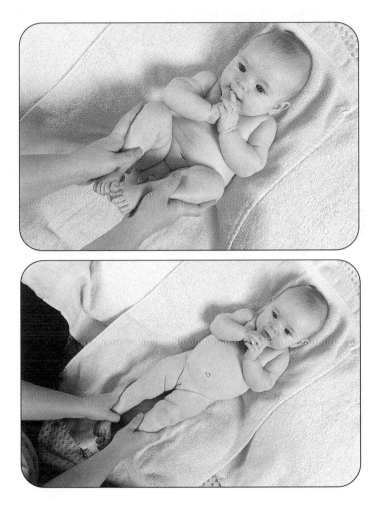

b) Then pull the knees together up into the abdomen and stretch them out straight.

c) Pull the knees together up into the abdomen and rotate round each way to help gently massage the baby's lower back.

Note If the baby resists any of the stretches, advise the parent to gently shake the limb to encourage relaxation.

NB. It is imperative that if the baby has any joint problems, that stretches are **NOT** undertaken and medical advice is sought as to their suitability.

Additional Baby Massage Techniques

As babies develop, parents will want to introduce additional techniques and different positions to add variety to the session.

Most of the techniques illustrated in the 5-minute routine may also be carried out in a seated position once the baby is able to sit up, as illustrated below:

Connecting strokes to the front of the body with baby in a seated position ▼

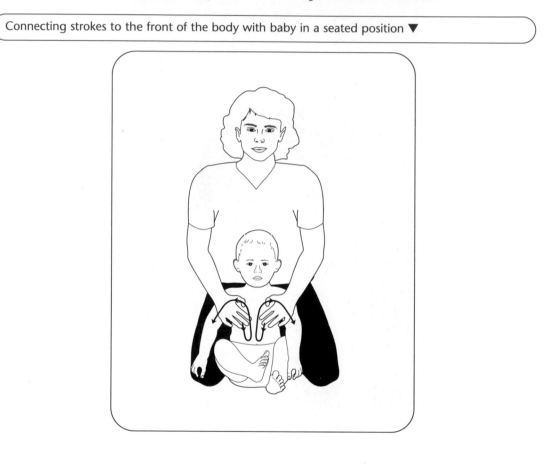

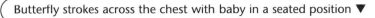

Butterfly strokes across the chest with baby in a seated position ▼

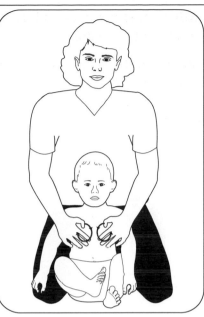

Massage of the abdomen with baby in a seated position ▼

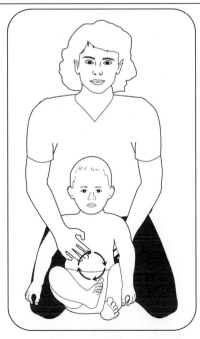

Note When the baby is in this position, it is an ideal opportunity to massage the chest, arms, the abdomen and the legs.

Connecting stroke to the back of the body with baby in a seated position ▼

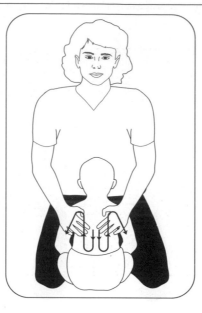

Note When the baby is in this position it is an ideal position for massaging the back, arms and the legs.

The following techniques may be carried out when the baby is either lying down or sitting up, on the floor or on the parent's/carer's lap.

Figure of 8

1   Figure of 8 movements across the whole of baby's back. Repeat × 6.

Figure of 8 across the back with baby in a seated position ▼

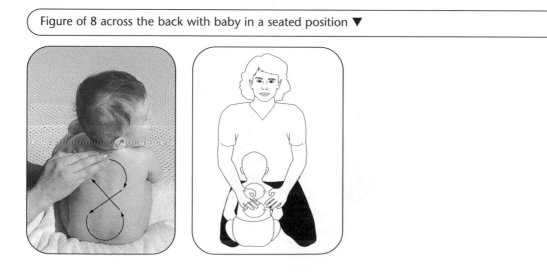

Rocking Movement to Base of Spine

2 Rock and gently massage the base of the baby's spine with the heel of the hand. Repeat × 3.

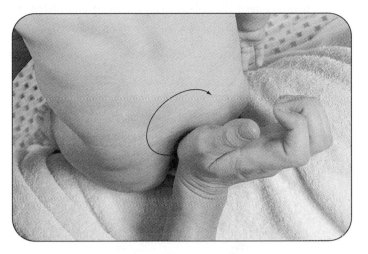

Caterpillar Walking

3 Caterpillar walking down either side of the baby's spine with the index and middle fingers. Repeat × 6.

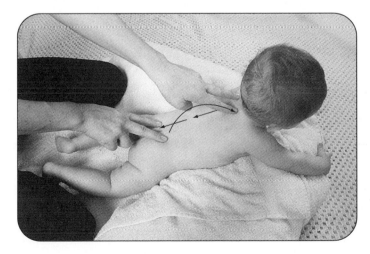

Lifting Side-to-Side

4 Lifting side-to-side across the back (if baby is lying down one hand is one side of the back and the other is on the other side), draw both hands up towards the spine lifting as you go and then slide back down the sides. Progress the strokes up and down the back. Repeat × 6.

NB. If carrying out this movement whilst the baby is sitting up one hand should be used to lift from side to side.

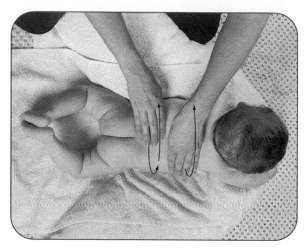

Tapping

5 Gentle tapping down the back with the tips of the fingers. Repeat × 3.

Baby Massage Techniques for the Face and Head

Some babies may initially resist massage of the head due to birth trauma and their temples may be tender for some time following delivery.

Parents and carers should take care to avoid pressing on the fontanelles when massaging the baby's head.

Facial massage may also initially seem a little too invasive to some babies.

The following techniques may either be carried out with the baby in a lying or seated position.

Stroking to the Temples

1 Gentle stroking to the temples with the pads of both ring or middle fingers. Repeat × 6.

Figure of 8 around the Eyes

2 Trace the ring or middle finger of one hand around the contours of the baby's eye in a figure of eight. Repeat × 3.

Figure of 8 around the Eyes ▼

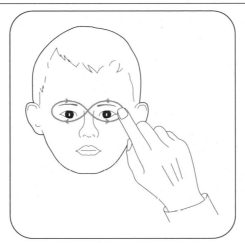

Gentle Pressures under the Eyebrow and Cheeks

3 Gently press and release under the eyebrow and then under the cheek bones. Repeat × 3.

Gentle Pressures under the Eyebrow and Cheeks ▼

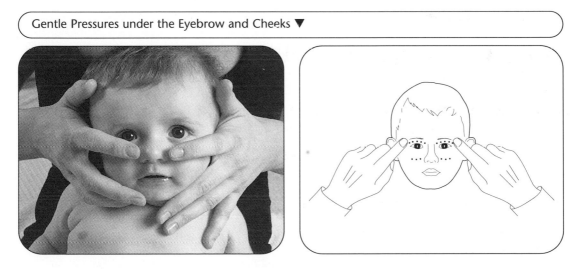

Sliding up the Bridge of the Nose

4 Slide the index or middle fingers of both hands alternatively up the bridge of the nose. Repeat × 6.

Sliding up the Bridge of the Nose ▼

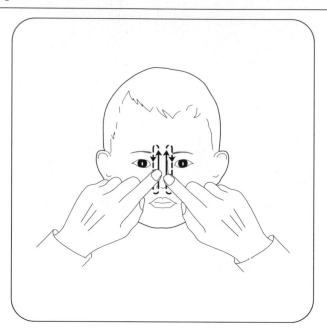

Gentle Squeeze of the Earlobes

5 Gently squeeze the lobes of the ears in between the thumbs and forefingers of both hands. Repeat × 3.

Circular Technique with the Palms to Baby's Temples

6 Using the heels of both hands on the sides of baby's temples, press in very gently and then circle × 3.

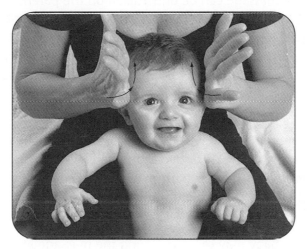

Summary of Guidelines for Massage for Babies of Different Ages

Baby's Age	Massage Guidelines
0–3 months	It is usual to massage a baby after an ample amount of weight has been gained and the post-natal check has been carried out. However, new-born babies enjoy having their heads and back lightly stroked and this is a good way for parents/carers to start massaging their babies. Massage is a sensory experience for a baby and can help young babies feel secure and develop sensitivity to touch. It is very important to be aware that babies of around 1 month, have little head control and underdeveloped muscle tissue. Bones are not fully ossified (cartilage in hands, fingers, feet and toes) so light pressure should be used. Mainly effleurage strokes will be used initially, usually with the ring and middle fingers and not the whole hand. The massage will usually be of a short duration and can be undertaken outside of a baby's soft clothing (e.g. baby's sleepsuit) as babies of this age dislike being undressed.

Baby's Age	Massage Guidelines
	The massage can be undertaken on the parent's lap due to the size of the baby as it offers additional closeness and support. As the baby's muscles develop and head control is established more variety may be added with stretching and mobility exercises. As babies become more alert it is a good time to introduce more movement into routines and to start adding songs and rhymes.
3–6 months	For a baby of 6 months, more pressure may be used and more variety of strokes added as the baby will have developed more muscle tissue. The baby may also sit for a while with support and therefore the massage strokes may be carried out in a seated position.
	The baby may roll over during the massage and parents should be encouraged to follow the baby's lead and not forcibly try to massage them in a certain position. Different positions may be tried to suit the baby's needs.
	Communication through touch can be reinforced by plenty of vocalisations through songs, nursery rhymes etc. Stretching and mobility exercises are an important feature of routines and the baby will begin to anticipate these so repetition is good.
6–9 months	Mobility becomes a challenge to massage sessions at this age.
	The length of limbs and density of tissue will allow for a firmer pressure to be used and a variety of techniques to be employed (deeper effleurage, petrissage and frictions).
	Music and rhymes are an important feature and will help to reduce boredom. Mobility exercises are still an important feature. The massage may be of longer duration but may have to be shortened due to tolerance levels.
	It may be helpful to suggest massage is undertaken before bedtime when the baby is less active, thereby encouraging relaxation and sleep.

Baby's Age	Massage Guidelines
9–12 months	At this stage the baby may be crawling, pulling themselves to standing, or walking! Mobility continues to present a challenge to massage sessions (massage at this age is usually most effective as part of a bedtime routine).
	Playing games and singing songs and rhymes that involve touch, smiles, cuddles, kisses and smiles all help to reinforce the massage session as fun and lots of repetition will encourage learning and communication skills.
	The massage session is no longer so structured and may involve more movement/soft gymnastics to aid the baby's development and add interest. If the baby is resistant to massage, encourage parents to find other ways for closeness (cuddles etc).
12–15 months	Mobility continues to present a challenge although most babies who have been massaged regularly will anticipate the sessions and look forward to them (particularly if it is around the same time of day).
	There may be a 'battle of the wills' as the baby starts to assert independence by increasing mobility. Advise parents to learn from their baby's cues as to which strokes they favour and which they dislike. Mobility exercises/soft gymnastics help a baby to develop flexibility and encourage relaxation.
15–18 months	Babies of this age may enjoy imitating massage strokes; through this they learn that positive touch is part of everyday life. Massage shown on their favourite teddy may promote them to want to experience the same.
	Massage may need to be shorter in duration, due to tolerance levels and the baby's increasing strive for independence. If the baby resists massage on the body encourage parents to try massaging their head whilst seated, or massage their face whilst being cuddled before a sleep.
	Babies of this age often enjoy their feet and hands being massaged whilst they are sitting on their parent's/carer's lap.

The Challenge of Massaging Twins

Parents with twins (or more) will have extra challenges when caring for their babies, and they may feel it impossible to integrate massage into their already hectic schedule! When preparing to massage twins, it is simply a case of finding a different way of approaching it.

It is usually best to try to encourage parents to involve another family member to make the session more of a family experience. If there is an older child in the family then they could be encouraged to be included.

Considerations for massaging twins include the following:

* each individual baby is likely to have different needs
* each individual baby may respond to being massaged at a different time of day to the other twin.

Common Baby Ailments and How Baby Massage Can Help

Colic and Wind

Colic is a very common problem for babies less than 4-months-old. Colicky pains are due to waves of contraction in the muscles of the intestine. In the first few months, some babies seem to have colicky abdominal pains following feeds, particularly after the evening one. They have a high-pitched distressed cry and draw their legs up and go red in the face indicating pain.

The crying spell can last between one and three hours during which the baby will not usually stop as a result of the parent/carer's normal methods of soothing.

Abdominal massage can be very useful for colic and trapped wind, as well as the leg stretches illustrated on page 173.

It is worth pursuing with these techniques for several weeks as it may take some time before there will be a significant improvement. The upright holding position is also useful for helping to provide relief from colic or wind. Stand holding your baby upright against your chest with his or her back to you. Place one arm round baby's abdomen, below the ribs for support. Place your other hand over the nappy and between the thighs. You can either walk around or rock and bounce your baby gently on the point. This position usually helps to bring up wind and relieve the pain in the baby's stomach.

Prone suspension is a comforting holding position for many infants. The parent/carer holds their baby to them and brings the left arm under to support the baby's chest (baby cradles their head into crook of parent elbow) and the right hand is placed between the baby's knees with the palm placed flat over the baby's tummy.

The gravity in combination with the baby's body weight over the parent/carer's hand produces slight pressure into the baby's abdomen. This holding may be combined with gentle clockwise movements to the abdomen or with a slight backwards and forwards movement.

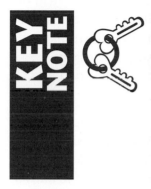

KEY NOTE

Useful dietary advice for breast-feeding mothers is to avoid dairy products, chocolate, caffeine, citrus fruits and spicy foods. When nursing a colicky baby try eliminating all gas-producing foods from your diet, including broccoli, beans, onions, peppers, cauliflower, brussels sprouts and cucumbers.

Useful advice for bottle-fed infants is to feed babies more often with smaller amounts and offer bottled water between feeds.

Constipation

Most babies have two or three bowel actions a day. The stool is soft and the baby does not have to strain to pass it. However, breast-fed babies have much less frequent stools, either once a day or even every two days. The reason for this is that the milk may be so well absorbed that there is little residue to be passed. Constipation is much more common in bottle-fed babies. Stools are infrequent and hard and the baby has to strain, which causes discomfort.

Babies who are constipated generally respond to gentle massage over the abdominal area in a clockwise direction, and to gentle stretching movements of the legs.

These techniques can just as easily be performed over the clothes (my daughter now asks me to rub her tummy when she is constipated or has a tummy ache).

It is also important for parents to ensure their baby is drinking enough fluids and that there is enough fibre in their diet to help relieve or prevent constipation.

Coughs and Colds

Babies often suffer with repeated coughs, cold and congestion due to the fact that they are initially 'mouth breathers'.

Massaging your baby's chest and upper back can help to loosen phlegm and expel excess mucus, which block the airways.

The sinuses and nostrils can be cleared by gently pressing either side of your baby's nostrils and under the cheekbones.

Babies benefit from being propped up more when congested, so use a soft pillow on your lap to have your baby facing you at the same height as your face.

Eczema

Eczema is an allergic skin condition which produces an itchy, dry, scaly red rash on face, neck, limbs, trunk and in the creases of the limbs. Sometimes other areas can be involved, and if severe the whole body can be affected. At first the rash may show small blisters which weep clear fluid if scratched. As a result of the baby scratching and chronic inflammation the skin often becomes dry, thickened and scaly.

The most common form of eczema in babies is atopic eczema, which usually develops when a baby is about 2 to 3 months, or around 4 to 5 months when solid foods are introduced. Although a tendency to develop is hereditary the skin can be made worse by allergy either to something that comes into contact with the baby's skin, such as soap or certain clothing, or to certain types of food, commonly dairy products, eggs and wheat.

An eczema attack can also be triggered by stress or an emotional upset.

Another form of eczema, known as seborrhoeic eczema, commonly occurs on the scalps of babies (cradle cap), on the eyelashes and eyelids (blepharitis), in the external ear canal (otitis externa) and in the greasy areas around the nostrils, ears and groin. Seborrhoeic eczema is not as itchy as atopic eczema.

Provided the eczema is not too inflamed, sore and the skin is unbroken, gentle massage with a suitable anti-inflammatory oil (such as calendula or jojoba) can be beneficial as it will help to moisturise the skin as well as soothe the skin and the baby.

Fractious Crying

Babies typically cry when they are hungry, tired, over-stimulated, need a change of position or scenery, need a cuddle, or are in pain.

Babies cry on average for around two hours a day; parents or carers soon learn to distinguish between different types of crying and know how to remedy the problem.

More distressing to the parent/carer is the baby who cries in obvious distress but without apparent cause and continues to cry despite being attended to.

Parents may feel on edge due to their baby's incessant crying, as it is impossible for them to relax or get on with other things, and they are possibly concerned about the constant noises upsetting the neighbours.

When parents become anxious or annoyed, the baby senses it and tends to react by becoming tenser and less likely to relax and the crying continues. It is therefore important for parents and carer to try to stay calm.

Many babies respond to being held and rocked and may feel happier being close to their parents/carers. Babies are often soothed by rhythmical sounds and it may be beneficial to play a special CD or tape designed for relaxing babies (see Resource section at the end of this book).

Although it is not normally recommended to commence massage whilst your baby is crying, massage may help to calm your baby between bouts of crying to help familiarise him or her with the idea of massage as a calming technique when he or she is feeling upset.

The most effective strokes for soothing a fractious baby are the long smooth flowing strokes which are performed rhythmically and slowly to reduce stress and anxiety.

Sleeping Problems

Sleeplessness can be a problem for many parents when their babies are very young, and can be more harmful for the parents than the child.

Babies vary in their sleep requirements from 18 to 20 hours daily to as little as four or five hours!

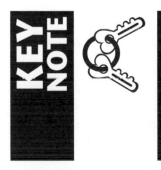

KEY NOTE

Babies have distinctly different sleep patterns to adults. Adults are in deep sleep for 75–80 per cent of the time and 20–25 per cent of the time in the shallow sleep cycle known as REM (rapid eye movement).

Newborn babies are half the time in deep sleep and half in shallow REM sleep. This explains why babies wake more easily and more often than older children and adults.

The key to successful sleep habits for babies and children of all ages is a sound pre-sleep routine. The bedtime routine is one of the most important you can establish.

When a baby begins to recognise their routine, they will relax and feel secure, knowing what to expect.

The important thing is to choose a night-time ritual that your baby enjoys and one which comforts him or her. A relaxation tape or CD will help your baby to associate the massage sessions with relaxation.

This is where massage can be very beneficial, especially if combined with a bedtime routine i.e. bath, massage, bottle and bed. By developing a routine your baby will anticipate and expect what comes next and his or her experience of massage will be associated with sleep. Most babies fall into a deep and long sleep after a warm bath and a soothing massage.

Teething

The eruption of the teeth through the gum is often painful to babies and can give rise to restlessness, irritability and excess salivation. Much of the excess saliva is swallowed and may cause slight looseness of the bowels.

Gentle soothing massage of the hands and feet, and stroking across the back whilst cuddling a baby can help to reduce irritability whilst teething due to the stimulation of endorphins which help to relieve pain and may elevate the baby's mood.

Some babies may get temporary relief from teething by gently massaging the cheeks along the gum lines, although if the gums are very swollen the gentlest touch may feel uncomfortable. Most babies just want to be comforted and held when teething.

Common Reactions and Outcomes of Baby Massage

Alert—some babies may feel quite alert due to the stimulation of the massage. This may also be determined by the speed at which the strokes had been performed, or the time of day the massage is carried out.

Sleepy—many babies feel sleepy either throughout or towards the end of a massage, particularly if it is performed close to their regular sleep time (i.e. after a bath). Many parents report that their babies sleep longer and deeper after a massage.

Happy—many babies find massage an enjoyable experience and will coo, babble, smile and gurgle throughout the massage to express their pleasure. This helps to increase parental confidence and self-esteem and make the massage a very pleasurable experience for both parent and baby.

Unhappy—some babies may appear unhappy throughout or after the massage and this may simply be because they are tired, hungry or over-stimulated. Parents should be encouraged to read their baby's cues throughout the massage and not to become despondent if their baby appears unresponsive at the time. It is often simply that it is not a good time for massage, and parents should be encouraged to comfort and hold their baby and try again later.

Crying helps babies to communicate how they are feeling, and can be a form of healthy release, in that the baby may be releasing pent-up anguish. Some babies take three or four sessions before they become accustomed to massage and therefore it is worth parents persisting and introducing a few strokes little by little until their baby becomes familiar with the strokes and the sensations experienced.

Hungry—it is advisable for parents to massage their babies in between feeds, because if their baby is hungry at the start of the massage he or she is unlikely to tolerate the massage session for long. Some babies will feel hungry and/or thirsty either throughout or after the massage and parents may be encouraged to stop and feed, or give their babies a drink either during or after the massage.

After Care Advice

Parents should be advised of after care advice following the massage session. It is particularly useful to the parent if the information is specified on a leaflet, which they may take home for future reference.

Parents should be advised to:

* cleanse their hands to remove all residual oil/massage medium before moving/dressing their baby
* remove any residue of oil/massage medium from their baby's skin after the massage, particularly if repositioning or bathing directly afterwards
* avoid exposing the baby to direct sunlight after the massage, as the oil on the skin could cause burning
* ensure that the baby is kept warm after the massage by wrapping them up in a warm towel or blanket
* ensure the baby has plenty of fluids after the massage, as the massage may make them feel hungry and thirsty (either cooled boiled water or prepared feed)
* allow the baby to sleep or relax after the massage if they want to, as the effects of the massage may make them tired
* monitor the baby's response to the massage.

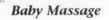

Frequency of Baby Massage

Parents will need to be advised how often to massage their babies. Ideally, a baby will benefit most by receiving a daily massage, if possible, for the first six months, and as the child becomes more active, the frequency may be reduced to once or twice a week.

However, frequency may be largely dependent on the baby's tolerance and the parent's schedule. Parents should be encouraged to experiment with different times of the day to find out which one works best for them and their baby. For younger babies a popular routine with parents is to massage their baby and then fill a warm bath, when the parent and baby can relax afterwards together.

From 6 months onwards, when bathtime becomes more of a playtime, the massage generally works better after the bath, when the baby is tired and ready for a nap.

Some parents may however want to massage their babies before they take a nap in order to help them sleep more soundly.

Evaluating Feedback from Parents and Babies

Feedback may be evaluated from parents and their babies in several ways.

A useful resource when conducting individual or group instruction is to ask parents to complete a pre-prepared parental feedback form.

See the example shown below:

Baby Massage Instruction—Parental Feedback Form

Please complete this evaluation form to help your Baby Massage Instructor ensure that you have received all relevant information necessary.

Baby's Name: _____

Parent /Guardian:_____

Instructor: _____

Were all the instructions you received clear, concise and informative?

Yes ( )   No ( )

Comments _____

Were you given sufficient time to ask questions?

Yes ( )   No ( )

Comments _____

Did you fully understand how to massage your baby using the relevant massage strokes?

Yes ( )   No ( )

Comments _____

Are there any areas which you are unsure about?

Yes ( )   No ( )

Comments _____

How do you feel about massaging your baby? _____

_____

_____

Please indicate your experience of learning baby massage.

	Low									High
Enjoyable	1	2	3	4	5	6	7	8	9	10
Helpful	1	2	3	4	5	6	7	8	9	10
Interesting	1	2	3	4	5	6	7	8	9	10

Do you have any other comments? _____

_____

_____

Signed:_____ Parent/Guardian

It is important for instructors to bear in mind that parents will tend to rate the effectiveness and enjoyment of the session based largely on their baby's response at the time of the instruction. If they can see their baby is responding and benefiting from the massage, then that will encourage them to continue at home.

It is more challenging for an instructor to encourage a parent to continue massaging when their baby is unresponsive, or becomes distressed during the massage. A parent may interpret this experience as negative and it may influence whether the massage is pursued further, and will most certainly affect the quality of the feedback given to the instructor.

A sensitive instructor will try to encourage the parent to continue to try to turn a potentially negative response into a more positive experience for a future session when the baby is more responsive and the time and setting is more appropriate.

Feedback may also be evaluated by the non-verbal signs of the parents and the baby.

The effectiveness of the massage session may be evaluated by observing the following throughout the massage:

* The degree of interaction and eye contact between parent and baby.
* The postures of the parent and baby (do they look comfortable and relaxed?).
* The quality and quantity of feedback given (verbal and written).
* The willingness of the parent/carer to continue with the massage at home.

Questions for Review

1. State the benefits of the following movements used in baby massage

    i) effleurage

    _____
    _____
    _____
    _____

    ii) petrissage

    _____
    _____
    _____
    _____

    iii) gentle stretching/joint movements

    _____
    _____
    _____
    _____

2. Outline the general guidelines and adaptations for babies of the following ages

    i) 0–3 months

    _____
    _____
    _____
    _____
    _____
    _____

ii) 3–6 months

_____
_____
_____
_____
_____
_____
_____

iii) 6–9 months

_____
_____
_____
_____
_____
_____
_____

iv) 9–12 months

_____
_____
_____
_____
_____
_____

3. Explain how massage may help babies and their parents with the following

i) colic

_____

_____

_____

_____

ii) constipation

_____

_____

_____

_____

iii) sleeping problems

_____

_____

_____

_____

iv) teething

_____

_____

_____

_____

4. State three common reactions of babies to massage

_____

_____

_____

5. State two ways in which an instructor may obtain feedback from parents and babies as to the effectiveness of the massage session

_____

_____

_____

_____

6. State at least five points of after care advice which a parent should be advised of following a baby massage session

_____

_____

_____

_____

7. What recommendations can an instructor suggest for frequency and dura-tion of baby massage?

_____

_____

_____

_____

Massage for Babies with Special Needs

Massage for Babies with Special Needs

Baby massage is a very valuable skill that parents can use to provide positive benefits to babies with special needs, as well as their families.

Parents of babies with special needs may feel helpless and powerless about the development outcome surrounding their baby's birth, as they find themselves in a more passive role than expected due to possible medical intervention.

Massage can be a valued adjunct in helping parents to care for their child with special needs, as it gives parents a positive tool to assist their child's development, as well as providing emotional support in helping with bonding and adjusting to their baby's needs.

This chapter gives an overview of special care conditions as well as the adaptations and other factors to be considered.

By the end of this chapter you will be able to relate the following knowledge to your role as instructor/parent/carer:

Baby massage adaptations for special care conditions including:

* premature babies
* autism
* cerebral palsy
* cystic fibrosis
* Down's syndrome
* muscular dystrophy
* sensory impairments
* spina bifida.

Premature babies—it is imperative for parents to seek medical advice before massaging their premature baby due to their fragile state.

Any form of massage given will naturally be limited by the small surface area of the pre-term baby, the immaturity of the baby's organs and the presence of any medical equipment.

An important consideration is that premature babies' bodies will have been traumatised and areas which may be sensitive include the feet, chest and head.

It may be possible for parents to introduce gentle stroking and hand placement whilst the premature baby is in the neonatal intensive care unit and then continue the relaxation at home to help release the trauma and tension of the hospital environment.

Premature babies may respond to touch and gentle massage most favourably on an area that has been least invaded by equipment (such as the back.) Parents can be encouraged to miniaturise each stroke and use a gentle pressure initially and monitor the baby's response.

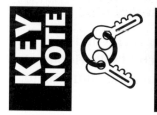

KEY NOTE

It has been proven in practice that premature babies respond positively to gentle stroking and massage as it helps encourage their growth and development, facilitates bonding that has been lost at the time of birth, as well as soothing and comforting the baby and its parents.

In Intensive Care Units babies are handled frequently as part of essential daily medical care and this can be distressing to both the baby and the parents.

Baby massage and gentle stroking is therefore encouraged in the pre-term infant as touch has been found to have a profound effect on development.

Benefits include:

* increase in daily weight
* increased bonding
* increased alertness and behavioural maturation increases at a faster rate
* reduction in stress (massage helps to lower the levels of cortisol in the blood).

Massage is generally carried out on the pre-term infant once around 1000g of weight has been reached.

Areas to massage other than the back are usually the arms, legs and the head (areas such as the chest and abdomen are generally too sensitive due to medical intervention). The feet can also be highly sensitive due to medical procedure (insertion of needles for blood tests).

If it is not practical to carry out the massage outside of the incubator due to the baby being too sick to move, light stroking can be undertaken through the portholes of the incubator.

> **Parental Note**
>
> Due to a pre-term baby's fragile medical state it is important to avoid over stimulation through massage and introduce gentle stroking slowly and monitor the baby's behavioural cues.

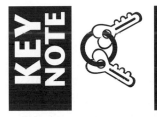

An important consideration when dealing with a baby or child with special needs is that they may have a sensory impairment in that they may be insensitive or highly sensitive to touch. It is important therefore to closely watch the baby's cues and adjust the pressure used accordingly.

Autism—this condition usually occurs from birth and is where a child has difficulty in relating to other people and making sense of the social world.

Autism is a spectrum disorder in which the symptoms and characteristics can present in a variety of combinations and with varying degrees of severity.

Autism affects a child's social interaction and communication; an autistic child may lack awareness of other people and have a problem with using non-verbal and/or verbal communication. They may also exhibit repeated body movements such as rocking or hand flapping.

Advise parent to seek their GP's advice before proceeding with massage.

It is important to remember that children with autism may overreact to many sensory input including sound, light, touch, smell etc. This is significant in the provision of massage. Massage may benefit a child with autism in calming and reducing anxiety in stressful situations. Benefits may include improved vocalisation, improved eye contact and attention which may be noticed during or after the massage.

Cerebral palsy—this is a disorder in which the part of the brain that controls movement and posture is damaged or fails to develop. Cerebral palsy covers a wide range of impairment in which there may be the following:

* **Spasticity**—where movements are stiff, muscles are tight and limbs are held rigidly and turned in towards the body
* **Athetosis**—where the limbs are floppy and movements are frequent and involuntary
* **Ataxia**—poor co-ordination and lack of balance.

Advise parents to seek advice from the GP/Physiotherapist concerning the baby's condition to ascertain whether massage is suitable.

Massage can help babies and children with cerebral palsy in the following ways:

* increasing muscle tone and co-ordination by improving the circulation to the affected muscle groups
* helping to reduce spasticity and prevent contractures
* improving posture
* helping with digestion and respiration.

An important consideration when dealing with a baby or child with cerebral palsy is that they may have a sensory impairment in that they may be insensitive or highly sensitive to touch. It is important therefore to closely watch the baby's cues and adjust the pressure used accordingly.

Cystic Fibrosis (CF)—this is a hereditary and life-threatening condition that affects the lungs and the digestive system. It is a recessively inherited condition and for the child to be affected, both parents must carry the CF gene.

It involves breathing difficulties, coughing and repeated chest infections due to the presence of thick and sticky mucus through the airways and into the lungs.

Advise the parent to consult the GP concerning massage for their child. The aim of massage in a child with cystic fibrosis would be to help drain the viscous mucus from the lungs and to increase the blood flow and lymph drainage in the fatigued respiratory muscles.

NB: As children with this condition are prone to respiratory infection, it is important to ensure that they do not come into contact with any form of infection.

Down's Syndrome—this condition is caused by an abnormal chromosome that affects the child's appearance and development. Children with Down's syndrome have 47 chromosomes instead of the normal 46 in each cell.

The condition may be identified soon after birth by the presence of typical characteristics. Not all children will show all characteristics to the same degree, but they may include some of the following:

* short hands and feet
* poor muscle tone
* small jaw: tongue appears large
* almond-shaped eyes
* poorly developed nose, sinuses and lungs with increased susceptibility to infections.

Parents should be encouraged to consult the baby's GP; approximately 50 per cent of Down's syndrome children have a heart defect, and a smaller number are born with a blockage in the intestine.

However, massage is usually recommended as it may help to aid relaxation, aid digestion, increase the tone of muscles and improve balance and co-ordination.

As Down's children generally have a love of music and rhythmic games, the massage schedule may be adapted to incorporate this into the routine.

Muscular Dystrophy (Duchenne)—this is a life-threatening condition involving progressive destruction of muscle tissue. The condition only affects boys, as it is an abnormality of the X chromosome inherited through the female.

Advise parents to seek their GP's advice before proceeding with the massage and to exercise caution as muscles will be painful.

The effects of massage can be positive in that may help to slow down muscle atrophy, and lightly massaging over the abdominal area may help with constipation due to the effect of the disorder on the involuntary nervous system.

Spina Bifida—this is a congenital defect in which the lower part of the spine, and often the spinal cord, does not develop fully, so that at a birth a defect is present in the lower back. It involves a defect in the fusion of the right and left half of one or more vertebrae during the development of the foetus, resulting in malformation of the spine. There may or may not be protrusion of the spinal cord and meninges through the gap.

There are two main forms of spina bifida:

spina bifida occulta, in which the skin is intact; this rarely causes disability

spina bifida cystica, which has two types:
* Meningocele, where there is a fluid-filled sac on the back, where the fluid and membranes of the spinal cord protrude through the gap in the bones of the spine

* Mylomeningocele, in which the sac contains spinal fluid and the nerves of the spinal cord. This is the most severe form and there will be some degree of paralysis below the spinal defect.

Advise the parent to seek their GP's advice before proceeding with massage.

It is important for parents to consider that with spina bifida the damage may be partial, with variable loss of power and sensation below the spinal defect. In severe cases the legs, bladder and bowel may be totally paralysed and sensation absent over the legs.

However, the provision of gentle massage can help to promote circulation, aid digestion, maintain skin integrity, enhance existing sensation, as well providing visual awareness of the lower extremities.

Sensory Impairments

Hearing Impairments

Hearing impairments fall into two main categories:

Conductive deafness—an interruption to the mechanical process of conducting sound through the ear drum and across the middle ear.

Nerve deafness—damage to the cochlea, the auditory nerve or the hearing centres in the brain.

The range of impairment is very wide, from slight loss to profound deafness.

Causes of hearing impairment include:

* heredity
* impairment of the cochlear nerve of the inner ear
* maternal rubella during pregnancy
* congenital defects
* head injury
* middle ear infection (otitis media)
* infections such as meningitis
* toxic action of some drugs (such as streptomycin)
* blockage of the ear canal by wax or other foreign bodies.

When massaging a child with a hearing impairment, the following guidelines should be considered.

✳ It is essential for parents to maintain eye contact at all times throughout the massage and carefully observe the baby's cues to determine responsiveness and tolerance.

✳ It is important to provide the baby with many visual cues throughout the massage.

✳ Decrease any background noises to enable the baby to concentrate on the focus of the massage and the intent of the movements.

✳ For older babies and children, the massage strokes may be demonstrated on another child or doll, and sign language may be used throughout to explain the procedure.

Visual Impairments

Visual impairment may be present at birth or may occur later. There are two main categories of visual impairment—blind or partially sighted.

The causes of congenital blindness include infections in pregnancy such as rubella and syphilis, optic nerve atrophy or tumour. Causes after birth include cataract, glaucoma and infections such as measles and the herpes virus.

Massage can be a very effective way to encourage interaction with a baby or child who has a visual impairment.

Massage is a universal form of communication and through touch parents can help their child to feel secure and to form meaningful associations with sounds, smells and sensations.

When massaging a child with a visual impairment it is important to:

✳ explain the process carefully; the intonation of the parent's/carer's voice is very important as it assists the baby in learning to anticipate change by talking before touching or repositioning

✳ describe the body parts being massaged; this will help a visually impaired child to develop a body image

✳ let the child explore the resources used for the massage (massage oil bottle, your hands)

✳ carefully observe the baby's cues and the baby's body language to determine responsiveness

❊ decrease any background noises to enable the baby to concentrate on the focus of the massage and your voice

❊ hold and cuddle your baby frequently throughout to offer reassurance and a feeling of security.

Questions for Review

1. Why is it beneficial to encourage parents of babies with special needs to massage their babies?

    _____

    _____

    _____

    _____

2. State the considerations for massaging

    i) a baby who is premature

    _____

    _____

    _____

    _____

    _____

    _____

    ii) a baby with cerebral palsy

    _____

    _____

    _____

    _____

    _____

    _____

    iii) a baby with a visual impairment

    _____

    _____

    _____

    _____

    _____

    _____

iv) a baby with an autism/autistic spectrum disorder

_____

_____

_____

_____

_____

_____

Baby Massage Instruction 11

Baby Massage Instruction

A baby massage instructor should start out with a different approach than when carrying out a massage with a client; what happens between a parent and their child is different from what happens during a therapeutic massage—the act of bonding.

The skill of an instructor is to gently guide the parent throughout the massage but aim to empower them in order that they may feel confident to carry out the massage at home, as part of the ongoing physical and emotional nourishment for their baby.

By the end of this chapter you will be able to relate the following knowledge to your role as an instructor:

❋ Qualities of a good baby massage instructor

❋ Preparation for an Instruction Session—an Instructor's Checklist

❋ Considerations for Group Instruction and Individual Instruction

❋ Instruction Session Planning—Teaching and Learning Objectives

❋ Teaching resources and aids

❋ Timing of the Instruction Session

❋ Factors for Instructors to consider when conducting classes.

Qualities of a Good Baby Massage Instructor

❋ Calm and relaxed manner—able to put parents at their ease

❋ Plenty of patience

❋ Friendly, positive and approachable

❋ Good communication skills and ability to listen actively (to verbal and non-verbal signs)

* Supportive of parents and their parenting styles (non-judgmental)
* Clear vocal instruction—well paced, relaxing and calm with intonation/reinforcement
* Ability to give positive encouragement of parent's innate abilities (even when session is not going as planned!)
* Flexibility—needs to be able to adapt the session according to the needs of parent/baby
* Ability to act as facilitator and avoid 'taking over'
* Good preparation and time management skills.

Preparation for an Instruction Session—an Instructors Checklist

When planning an instruction session, it is essential to have a checklist to ensure that the instructor has all the necessary resources to hand, particularly as the instruction is likely to involve the instructor travelling to an agreed venue.

* Visual aids (baby dolls, basic illustrations of massage movements, posters etc).
* Promotional/information leaflets on baby massage (with instructor's contact details on).
* Suitable oils/lotions/creams.
* Dry hand cleansers.
* Wipes and tissues.
* Consultation forms, treatment records and parental feedback forms.
* Cushions and pillows.
* A few soft baby toys.
* CD player and music CD/tape.

It is advisable to prepare an explanatory leaflet that may be given out to the parents prior to, or during, the introductory sessions which may include information such as:

* benefits and effects of baby massage to baby and parents
* hygiene and safety precautions
* occasions when it may not be safe to massage your baby
* an outline guide to the massage sequence
* after care advice.

Considerations for Group Instruction and Individual Instruction

Group Instruction

❋ The number of participants (from experience I have found it is best to stick to a maximum of six in a group to maximise interaction).

❋ Checking out the venue and its suitability i.e. is it parent-friendly and the right setting (check size, accessibility, hygiene/cleanliness, health and safety, lighting power supply, heating, parking, comfort, mother and baby rooms, refreshments etc).

❋ The layout for instruction—it is ideal if there is enough room to have the instructor seated in the middle of the group, with parents side by side (this avoids anyone having to interpret and follow the instruction from an upside-down position).

❋ Giving parents a checklist of items they need to bring with them prior to the session (always bring spares in case someone forgets).

❋ Having enough resources to go round (oils etc).

❋ Consultations and whether these may be undertaken before the instruction session to save time (check for any contra-indications).

❋ Consider timing carefully, as it will take longer with a group due to the fact that not all babies will adhere to the proposed schedule!

❋ The ages of the babies in the groups (it is important to have this information beforehand as it will enable the instructor to be as prepared as possible). Classes with mixed aged babies will need different instruction.

❋ It is useful to have an extra pair of hands to help set up/pack up at the end/help with refreshments and therefore it is handy to take a friend or colleague with you.

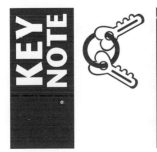

KEY NOTE

When carrying out a group instruction it is very important to consider the positioning of the instructor carefully. The best position is to have parents and their babies encircled around the instructor (who is positioned in the centre) to ensure everyone can focus on the instruction. This also ensures parents can mirror the instructor's strokes and not be confused by an upside-down image.

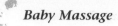
Individual Instruction

As the individual instruction session will usually take place in the parents' home, the instructor does not need to consider the venue and its suitability.

Considerations when instructing an individual include:

* Giving the parent/carer a checklist of items needed in order that they are prepared for when the instructor arrives.

* The place in the home to carry out the instruction (consider where there is sufficient space, safety etc; the parent may consider the bedroom too private and intrusive).

* Timing (allow additional time for the first session to allow for preparation of the instruction area etc).

* Other household distractions (is the instruction going to take place without interruptions?).

* Arrange the instruction for a suitable time with the parent to ensure it does not interfere with other regular routines the baby may have.

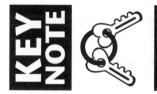

KEY NOTE

When carrying out an individual instruction it is best to be positioned to one side of the parent/baby.

Instruction Session Planning—Teaching and Learning Objectives

When preparing for an instruction session, always prepare an outline plan, with aims and objectives in order that you can pace the session and keep to the required allocated time.

An Example of a Baby Massage Instruction Session Plan

Duration: 1 hour

Aims

* to enable parents to understand the benefits of baby massage
* to enable parents to participate in providing massage to their babies.

Objectives

By the end of the session, parents will

❋ be able to identify and select different massage mediums for baby massage

❋ carry out a simple 5-minute routine on their babies.

Session Plan ▼

Outline of Contents	Parent/Carer Activity	Teaching Resources
5 minutes Introduction of instructor History and development of baby massage	Listening	Flipchart/OHP/ PowerPoint presentation Handouts (All items from instructor's checklist— oils, mats, pillows etc.)
10 minutes Benefits of baby massage	Listening Discussion with instructor	Flipchart/OHP/ PowerPoint presentation Handout Examples of successful case studies
10 minutes Consultation for baby massage (including when it is not advisable to massage baby)	Each parent to complete their baby's details, including medical checklist	Flipchart/OHP/ PowerPoint presentation Handout Consultation forms with parental consent
5 minutes Preparation for baby massage (including safety and hygiene precautions)	Instructor to demonstrate preparation; parents to prepare their area to massage and ensure they have all items to hand	Flipchart/OHP/ PowerPoint presentation Handout
5 minutes Discussion of suitable massage mediums for baby massage	Parents to choose medium suitable for their baby's skin	Flipchart/OHP/ PowerPoint presentation Handout

Outline of Contents	Parent/carer activity	Teaching Resources
15 minutes Demonstration of simple 5-minute baby massage routine on baby doll	Parents to watch demonstration and then mirror strokes with instructor demonstration	Live demonstration of massage strokes on baby doll Illustrations of baby massage strokes
5 minutes After Care Advice	Listening	Handout/Leaflet
5 minutes Feedback and questions	Q & A session	
Confirm date of next session		

Visual Aids and Teaching Resources

As baby massage is a practical skill, it is essential to have a variety of visual aids to help reinforce learning. It is important to remember when instructing that parents will have different ways of learning, and will have differing levels of experience and confidence.

When instructing the best visual aids include the following:

1 **Live demonstration** of the massage routine by the instructor on a baby doll—this is by far the most effective visual aid for effective instruction, as the demonstration can be paced to suit individual or group requirements. The pace of the demonstration needs to be carefully considered, as each technique will need to be miniaturised to facilitate learning.

2 **Illustrations of the baby massage routine**—these could be enlarged onto a large poster or board and displayed around the demonstration room to help reinforce the techniques, a smaller version could be given to parents in a leaflet format, which may also be taken away at the end. Useful factors to consider when giving out illustrations is whether they are the logical, easy to follow, large enough to read and most importantly do they show the direction of the stroke and an explanation of the techniques?

2 **Video**—a video is a useful learning aid; however it does not supplant the need for live demonstration. The disadvantage with a video for a group is that everyone will be working at different paces and it may be difficult for everyone to follow (remember parents' attentions will be diverted at times). A video would be useful

for parents to follow at home as they could play it and reinforce learning at their own pace.

Timing of the Instruction Session

If you have an individual to instruct, you may find that two or three sessions of approximately one hour may be enough for them to familiarise themselves with the techniques and gain confidence. If instructing a larger group, you may find that you will need four sessions of approximately one hour.

The first session will give the instructor an opportunity to familiarise herself or himself with the parents/guardians and their babies and for a consultation to be undertaken.

It will also give the parent/guardian an opportunity to ask any questions and for you to reassure them of any worries or fears they may have before starting.

After the consultation has been undertaken and you are ready to start the first session, this will generally involve a demonstration of a 5-minute massage routine which can be easily integrated into the busiest of home lives.

On the subsequent sessions, it will give the instructor and parents/guardians an opportunity to review the last sessions and the baby's response to the massage and how the parent felt.

The second session may require a review and recap of the 5-minute routine or the parent/guardian may feel confident to be shown additional techniques.

Before starting the massage session, it is important to reassure the parent/carer that although you will be demonstrating the techniques as a guide for them to follow, there is no right or wrong to massage.

If the baby responds favourably to a particular stroke, then they should be encouraged to repeat it and let their instinct and the baby's feedback guide them.

Guidance for Instructors

It is important for the instructor to allow the parent to develop their own style, thereby empowering them and not allowing them to turn over their power to the instructor as the 'expert'.

Instructors need to bear in mind that baby massage is an interaction that is done with the baby, rather than to the baby, and is therefore an experience that belongs to babies and their parents.

A baby massage instructor will generally use a doll to demonstrate the strokes and relational dynamics of the massage. Since the parent is the one who is massaging the baby, success is attributed to the parent's competence, rather than to the manual skills of either a therapist or the instructor.

Parental success will ensure the continuity of baby massage in the family, thereby deepening attachment and quality of family life.

Factors for Instructors to Consider when Conducting Baby Massage Instruction Classes

✳ Make the instruction as relaxed as possible; this will help increase learning and enjoyment of both parent and baby.

✳ Speak slowly and clearly with intonation in your voice—allow parents time to absorb what is being said as well as what is being demonstrated! (don't forget that they will also be concentrating on their baby's needs).

✳ Be aware of differing emotions of new parents; emotions may swing from elation to depression, guilt, anger, frustration and disempowerment to name a few!

✳ Try and build-in coping mechanisms for parental stress, offer helpful tips and advice for common problems (colic, sleeping problems etc) and offer advice for parents' well-being).

✳ Some parents may have little or no massage experience and may possibly harbour a negative bias around the issues of touch.

✳ It is important to maintain the sensitivity and regard for the parents' self-esteem and accept where they are in the parenting process. The role of the instructor is as a facilitator and should therefore be supportive.

✳ Allow parents to develop their own style—they know their baby better than anyone!

✳ Stress the need to adapt and offer flexibility. If difficulties are experienced suggest adaptations and different positioning in order to make the experience a positive one for them.

✳ If a massage movement or positioning is not effective, advise the parent not to forcibly hold their baby in that position but to find an alternative in accordance with the baby's needs.

✳ Work on building parental confidence as their success will ensure continuity of baby massage at home and within the family.

✳ Encourage parents to actively listen and respond to their babies' needs.

✳ Encourage parents to learn, watch and interpret their baby's reaction to touch. This will enable them to be in touch with their baby's natural rhythm, likes and dislikes.

Questions for Review

1. List five qualities of a good baby massage instructor

    _____
    _____
    _____
    _____
    _____
    _____
    _____

2. State three considerations for the following

    i) Group Instruction of Baby Massage

    _____
    _____
    _____
    _____
    _____
    _____

    ii) Individual Instruction of Baby Massage

    _____
    _____
    _____
    _____
    _____
    _____

3. Why is it important for instructors to allow parents to develop their own style of massage with their baby?

    _____

    _____

    _____

    _____

    _____

    _____

4. State two teaching aids that an instructor may use to teach baby massage to parents/carers

    _____

    _____

    _____

    _____

    _____

    _____

    _____

    _____

    _____

5. Discuss three additional factors for instructors to consider from a parent's perspective when conducting baby massage instruction classes

    _____

    _____

    _____

    _____

    _____

    _____

    _____

    _____

Promotion and Marketing of Baby Massage Instruction Sessions

Promotion and Marketing of Baby Massage Instruction Sessions

Baby massage instruction classes are a relatively new concept for parents and therefore it is essential for instructors to consider ways in which they can market their services effectively.

Marketing is about telling potential clients (parents and carers) what you have to offer and most importantly how it will benefit them and their families.

This chapter looks at the different ways in which baby massage may be promoted within the community in order to raise awareness of its benefits.

By the end of this chapter you will be able to relate the following knowledge to your role as an instructor:

❋ Where and how to advertise baby massage classes

❋ Planning a talk on baby massage instruction

❋ Example of a promotional leaflet on baby massage

Where and how to advertise

The very nature of baby massage is in itself a personal service and therefore it is essential for instructors to make themselves known personally to parents.

This can be achieved through various means.

Word of mouth

This is the most effective and least expensive form of advertising for promoting baby massage classes. Once an instructor has established a good reputation, a satisfied parent will automatically recommend the service to another parent.

It is therefore important for instructors to communicate with as many parents as possible in order to inform them about what they do and how it can help.

One very effective way of doing this is to work on the current client group and inform them that baby massage is being introduced (even if baby massage does not apply to them, they usually have a friend or family member who may be interested).

Building a Referral Network

This is one of the most successful and inexpensive ways of creating new business.

Current satisfied parents are one of the most effective means of advertising.

Referrals can be encouraged by:

* offering existing clients incentives to introduce new parents to use your service
* establishing links with other professionals by making yourself and what you do known to them (midwives, health visitors, parent and baby group leaders, breast-feeding counsellors, post-natal/antenatal yoga/fitness teachers).

Talks and Demonstrations on Baby Massage

Talks and demonstrations are an effective way of presenting baby massage to a targeted group and they usually work best when presented together.

Talks should be informative and educational in nature (they should tell potential parents how it will benefit them and their babies) and will help to break down barriers or pre-conceptions parents may hold about the baby massage.

Talks are better being limited to a maximum of 30–40 minutes, with time left to answer questions and to distribute promotional literature. The focus of the talk should be about identifying with and providing solutions to parents' needs (massage as a solution to helping with colic, sleeping problems, restlessness etc).

A useful checklist when preparing for talks is to:

* find out as much as possible about the target group before the talk (approx. age of babies, are they new parents?)
* confirm the number of people that will be attending
* check out the venue and its suitability
* plan out the talk with a basic outline format
* have a plentiful supply of literature to hand out
* prepare a list of possible questions you may be asked
* take some relaxation music to help create a relaxing ambience
* aim to involve the audience in the session (encourage questions)
* take your appointment book with you!

Outline of a Short Promotional Talk to Parents on Baby Massage

Below is an example of a basic format of a promotional talk lasting approximately 45 minutes.

Aims

❋ To increase parental awareness of the benefits of baby massage

❋ To demonstrate a few basic massage strokes used in baby massage instruction.

Objectives

By the end of the talk, parents will:

❋ have an understanding of the benefits of massage to both parent and baby

❋ know what to expect from an instruction session

❋ know how to contact the instructor to book individual/group instruction sessions.

Content	Approximate time allocation	Resources/Visual Aids needed
Introduction of the role of a baby massage instructor Introduction of instructor (background, qualifications, insurance and code of ethics)	5 minutes	Flip chart/OHP/PowerPoint Handout
Brief history of baby massage	5 minutes	Flip chart/OHP/PowerPoint Handouts
Benefits of baby massage to parents and babies (concentrating on main problems associated with babies)	10 minutes	Flip chart/OHP/PowerPoint Handouts Photos/testimonials of clients who have discovered benefits (NB. with their permission to use the material for promotion) Poster

Content	Approximate time allocation	Resources/Visual Aids needed
Demonstration of a few basic baby massage strokes	10 minutes	Baby doll and other resources used in baby massage (oil, mat, pillow/cushion, hand cleanser, wipes etc) Poster
Frequently asked questions	5 minutes	Handout on FAQs
Question time	5 minutes	
How to book an instruction session	5 minutes	Hand out business cards, promotional leaflets and vouchers

Advertising for Hostesses for Baby Massage Classes

An effective way for instructors to facilitate classes in their area is to advertise for parents to act as a host for their own baby massage class. Incentives are given to the host such as free instruction and baby products, as they provide the venue as well as the parents and babies.

This can be an excellent way of generating interest for small groups of individuals who meet regularly anyway as it is less interruption to their normal routine, and is held in the comfort of the host's home.

Local Parent and Baby Exhibitions

Local exhibitions are an effective way to communicate with lots of parents with similar needs in one place. It is a useful way of distributing brochures and leaflets and of persuading new clients to find out about baby massage classes.

The National Childbirth Trust (NCT) has events such as Nearly New Sales held locally and a good source of contact for meeting up with parents with babies/young children.

Community centres and the local papers are another good source of information for finding what's on and where.

Public Relations

This is a way for instructors to get their name in the public eye without actually paying for advertising.

There are a variety of ways in which it can be done.

❋ Offering a free talk and demonstration to groups in the community is an ideal way of marketing baby massage and helping to get your name and reputation established. Public interest in baby massage is increasing all the time and there are many groups that meet regularly who may be keen to hear from you (NCT first time mums groups, antenatal groups, post-natal groups, Parentcraft classes at the local hospitals, parent and baby groups). See talks and demonstrations (page 218).

❋ Sending information or news concerning your classes to editors of newspapers or magazines in the form of a news article. Every day editors and journalists are looking for stories and information to fill their newspapers or magazines. An important consideration when sending information to journalists is to only send information that is truly of interest to the community and their readers.

❋ Donating your time, money or products to a local children's charity. There are many charitable organisations that rely on donations each year to survive. An event linked to funding or sponsoring a charity would be a newsworthy article, as well as helping to meet the needs of the community.

Indirect Approach to Marketing and Promotion

There are several other methods of advertising or marketing which may be used in order to reach the potential clients you cannot reach in person and these include:

❋ adverts in mother and baby magazines or publications

❋ leaflets and promotional material

❋ website.

Advertising is about getting your message across. Important considerations when considering an advert for baby massage are:

❋ What do you want to say to potential clients?

❋ Who is your target audience? (Parents, midwives, health visitors, parent and baby group leaders).

❋ How you will communicate to them what you want to say.

A good advert should be easy to read and be written to

❋ touch parents' emotions

❋ be informative

❋ promote the service on offer

❋ raise awareness

❋ motivate the reader to act.

Examples of Effective Adverts for Baby Massage Classes

Example 1 of Baby Massage advert ▼

Looking for a Natural Solution to your Baby's Sleeping Problems/Colic?

Baby Massage is a loving art that is relaxing to both parent and baby.

Benefits include:

❋ **Reducing tension, restlessness and irritability**

❋ **Promoting relaxation and inducing deeper and longer sleep**

❋ **Aiding digestion and elimination (can help relieve colic and constipation)**

❋ **Encouraging muscular co-ordination and joint flexibility**

Small friendly classes held locally by Qualified Baby Massage Instructor

Interested in finding out more ?

Please telephone ....

Also available for talks and demonstrations to antenatal/post-natal groups

Example 2 of Baby Massage advert ▼

Are you a New Parent ?

Have you heard about the gentle art of Baby Massage ?

Bring your baby along to a baby massage class and experience the many benefits of this soothing and gentle technique. Techniques are simple and easy to learn and may be easily fitted into your daily routine with your baby.

Baby massage is a form of loving communication for you and your baby to experience together.

Baby massage has many benefits for parents and their babies including

❋ **Reducing tension, restlessness and irritability**

❋ **Promoting relaxation and inducing deeper and longer sleep**

❋ **Aiding digestion and elimination (can help relieve colic and constipation)**

❋ **Encouraging muscular co-ordination and joint flexibility**

Small friendly classes held locally by Qualified Baby Massage Instructor

The next class starts on _____ at

_____

To book your place, or to find out further details

Please contact ....

Also available for talks and demonstrations to antenatal/post-natal groups

Promotional Material for Baby Massage

When writing and designing promotional material the key to success is to write it as if you know the parent or carer personally. Choose words carefully in order that they strike a cord with parents.

Promotional material must be attractive enough to encourage parents/carers to read it and wording should be positive, direct and above all personal.

It is also important to use positive language and turn a negative statement (baby's sleeping problems/colic) into a positive one (how baby massage is going to help them).

Brochures and posters with a question and answer format can help clients to overcome their objections and visual aids can help to attract attention.

Activity

Design a promotional leaflet advertising baby massage instruction to parents.

Displaying Promotional Literature on Baby Massage

Consider other local establishments or businesses that deal with new parents and who may be in a position to influence new parents to attend a baby massage class (baby shops, maternity shops, local community centres, GP surgeries, hospital antenatal wards and units, local leisure centres that hold antenatal/post-natal fitness classes, local music classes for babies (see resource section at end of book).

Parent and Baby Publications/Directories

Parent and Baby directories are an effective way of advertising as they are targeted to the client group baby massage is aimed at.

The Baby Directory is a wonderful resource for parents and is the ideal place for instructors to advertise (see Resource section at the end of the book).

It is published in counties and therefore unlike national publications it can be targeted to the area(s) in which the instructor is carrying out classes.

The National Childbirth Trust publish a quarterly branch newsletter and this is another cost-effective way for instructors to get their message across.

Website

The internet is an excellent form of advertising as it is cost-effective, direct and the information is immediately accessible to parents in their own homes at any time of day!

Having a web page displaying information on baby massage and how to contact the instructor for classes are an effective way of raising awareness of baby massage within the community. A web page can be designed in the form of frequently asked questions format to address the most common questions asked by parents and carers.

Introduction to Other Complementary Therapies as an Aid to Baby Massage

Introduction to Other Complementary Therapies as an Aid to Baby Massage

As complementary therapies increase in popularity, there is a growing interest in the use of various modalities as a valuable adjunct to baby massage.

This chapter aims to give an overview of some of the popular therapies that are now recognised to be beneficial in infant health care, and which parents may find a useful resource to help with common childhood problems such as colic, sleep problems and birth trauma to name but a few.

At the end of this chapter you will be able to relate knowledge of the following therapies to your role as instructor/parent/carer:

* baby yoga
* flower remedies
* cranial osteopathy
* homeopathy
* Tui Na massage.

Baby Yoga

Baby yoga is a revolutionary way to enhance a baby's development, and is an exercise that parents can do with their babies. It is an extension of baby massage as it adds movement, rhythm and fun to the session.

By using gentle movements and rhythm a baby's physical and emotional development can be stimulated. Baby yoga offers physical stimulation including flowing postures, holding, movement, touch and voice.

Yoga helps to relieve common babyhood ailments and can help babies to sleep well and relieve colic. By integrating 5 or 10 minutes of yoga into a baby's routine it can stimulate and balance all systems of a baby's body. The walks, lifts, swings and balances in baby yoga can all become an integral part of a parent and baby's routine.

It helps to give parents confidence in handling their baby and is a lovely way for parents to relax together with their baby.

It also helps both parent and baby develop good posture, and can be an excellent way of mothers finding their balance after giving birth.

Cranial Osteopathy

Cranial osteopathy is a specialist technique use to manipulate the bones of the skull with a touch so light that it is both gentle, safe and non-invasive in the treatment of babies and children.

The human skull is made up of 26 bones that are not fixed but can move slightly.

When the bones of the skull move normally the cranial rhythm remains balanced, but any disturbance to the cranial bones can disturb the normal motion of the bones and alter the cranial rhythm and the functioning of other parts of the body.

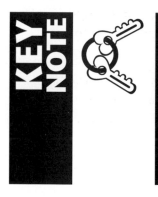

KEY NOTE

During labour and delivery, structures of the baby's body may become significantly compressed, resulting in a general decrease in function.

A trauma such as a difficult birth may cause a strain to the tissues, overstretching or compression. If the trauma is relatively small, the body may be able to heal itself. If it is moderate to large, the nervous system will contain the distortions and imbalances may appear.

A trained osteopath will feel the rhythm of the cranial pulse anywhere in the body, but principally at the skull and the sacrum. By holding and exerting very gentle pressure on the skull the practitioner can feel the rhythm of the cranial pulse and detect irregularities. The technique used in cranial osteopathy involves extremely gentle but specifically applied adjustments to the movement of body tissues. A cranial osteopath will gently 'listen' with their hands to detect little areas of tension and built up pressure that may be having a disturbing effect on a child.

There are many conditions that have been successfully treated by cranial osteopathy including asthma, co-ordination difficulties, dental problems, digestive problems, dyslexia, glue ear, hyperactivity, colic, sleeping problems, headaches and migraines.

Flower Remedies

This is a simple therapy that may be used to treat a child's emotional well-being.

Flower essences are simple and effective and may be used to:

* support in times of crisis
* treat the emotional symptoms produced by illness
* address a particular reoccurring emotional or behavioural pattern.

Flower essences work in a similar way to homeopathic remedies; they use the vibrational essence of the flowers to balance negative emotions that contribute to ill health.

Children are generally more expressive than adults and the emotions they show are often easily recognised and treated. Children and adults of all ages can benefit from them (they are safe to use for even the youngest babies).

Every flower essence has specific properties, and it is a case of choosing the most effective for your child. The flower remedies or essences bought in a shop are sold in single bottles but may be mixed in water to make a personal remedy for your child by combining up to five different remedies.

One of the Bach Flower Remedies, Rescue Remedy is a useful combination of five flower essences and can help babies, children and parents by soothing tension and irritability, easing fear and addressing the mental and physical symptoms of shock.

There are many other flower remedies that may be used according to your child's characteristics. Flower remedies may be purchased from a health food shop, or from some pharmacies.

Homeopathy

Homeopathy is one of the safest of all natural therapies, which makes it highly appropriate for use with babies and children. It is a gentle therapy, with no danger of toxicity or side-effects. Children seem to respond well to homeopathic remedies, probably due to the fact that they have fewer 'layers' to peel before the root cause becomes apparent.

Homeopathy is a system that supports the body's own healing, using specially prepared remedies. A homeopathic remedy is an extremely pure, natural substance that has been diluted many times.

Homeopathic remedies use plant and mineral bases and are prepared through a process known as 'potentisation' to bring out their subtle healing properties. The remedies help to rebalance the body's subtle energy system and once this is back in balance, the immune system and all the other interconnected systems in the body start functioning better.

There are thousands of homeopathic remedies that are sold in chemists and health food shops and it may be confusing to parents to choose the correct one for their child.

In order to get the correct remedy for your child, it is advisable to seek help from a trained homeopath.

Tui Na Massage for Babies

Tui Na is a unique form of healthcare that the Chinese have created to promote the development of a healthy body, a strong immune system, and a lively intellect during a child's formative years. It aims to strengthen and balance the internal organs to give a child resistance to disease and stimulation of the brain.

Fundamental to the traditional Chinese Medicine theory is the concept of Qi (Chi) that is the activating force for all life and flows within all living things. It is the flow and balance of Qi within a child's body that determines every aspect of development, health and potential. The flow of Qi can be affected by many physical factors such as exercise, sleep and diet, as well as the emotions. Disruptions to any of these factors results in either excesses or deficiencies.

Tui Na massage is a powerful method for restoring the balance of Qi and focuses on specific points where the flow of Qi may be manipulated, thereby restoring and promoting the free flow of Qi throughout the body.

Tui Na techniques may be used to help babies and children with common childhood problems such as colic, restlessness, coughs, colds and teething.

Frequently Asked Questions

Q. At what age should I start massaging my baby?

A. Babies may usually be massaged after their 6–8 week check, although it is perfectly natural for parents to want to use very light stroking movements from birth.

It is best to seek advice from a qualified baby massage instructor to check on your baby's individual suitability for massage.

Q. Is there any particular age when I should stop massaging my child?

A. No, follow your child's cues; if they want you to stop they will soon tell you.

When massaging an older child, the routine will need to be modified, however, as their needs will be different.

Q. Are there any reasons why I should not massage my baby?

A. Yes, there are several cautions, including if your baby has an infection, fever, or is generally unwell. There are other reasons why it may not be safe to massage your baby and these should be discussed with a baby massage instructor or advice sought from your baby's GP if you are unsure.

It is best not to massage your baby if they are hungry or very tired.

Q. How often can I massage my baby?

A. With a young baby, it is ideal if massage can be carried out as part of a daily routine. If this is not possible, try to integrate massage as often as you can, and most importantly in accordance with your babies needs and desires.

Q. How long should I massage my baby for, at any one time?

A. Once you are familiar with a simple routine, it can take around 5–10 minutes. Some babies will enjoy being massaged for longer, and will usually not tolerate longer than 20 to 30 minutes at any one time.

Q. What are the benefits of following a set routine?

A. Following a set routine will help your baby to anticipate what is next and besides, babies love routines and repetition.

Q. What equipment do I need to massage my baby with?

A. A few basics such as pillows, cushions, massage medium (if desired), a few soft towels, hand cleanser/wipes (it is best to have a prepared bottle or cooled boiled water near by for after the massage).

Q. Can I use essential oils to massage my baby?

A. It is best to avoid the use of essential oils in the first three months. It is advisable to seek advice from a qualified aromatherapist on the use of essential oils for babies of 3 months and above. There are several companies who supply proprietary brands of specially blended baby massage oils with essential oils. (See Resource section.)

Q. Where can I find oils/lotions to massage my baby?

A. You can find oils such as almond, sunflower, grapeseed, olive and jojoba in most health food stores. Please see the Resource section for suppliers of specially blended baby massage oils.

Q. What oils should I use if my baby has a nut allergy?

A. It is best to avoid any nut-based oils and stick to ones such as calendula, sunflower or grapeseed.

NB. Always patch test oils before using.

Q. Where can I find a qualified Baby Massage Instructor?

A. Please see the Resource section.

Q. I have a book and video on baby massage, is it still beneficial for me to attend a class?

A. Yes, absolutely as you will get so much more from a baby massage class. It will give you an opportunity to be guided personally by an instructor; you will have the opportunity to ask questions and to meet other parents.

Books and videos are very useful back-up resources once you have attended a baby massage course.

Resource Section

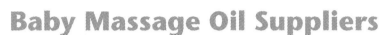

Baby Massage Oil Suppliers

Essensa UK
Distributed by
Helen McGuinness Health & Beauty
Abacus House
1 Spring Crescent
Portswood
Southampton
SO17 2FD
Tel: 02380 905545

Sells natural aromatherapy based baby products with no alcohol, no perfume or synthetics (made in Provence, France). The Essensa Baby massage emulsion is a beautiful massage medium for babies and children 3 months and over, and is a blend of essential essential oils including Sweet Orange, Pine, Petitgrain, Barreme Lavender, Eucalyptus, Rosewood, Palmarosa, Mandarin and Benzoin in an organic grapeseed base.

Neals Yard Remedies
UK shops in London, Brighton, Bristol, Bromley, Cardiff, Cheltenham, Edinburgh, Guildford, Manchester, Newcastle Upon Tyne, Norwich and Oxford.

Head Office
26–34 Ingate Place
Battersea
London
SW8 3NS
Tel: 020 7498 1686
E-mail: mail@nealsyardremedies.com

Neals Yard sells a baby massage oil (suitable for babies 3 months or over) which contains essential oils of Lavender, Roman Chamomile, Rose absolute and organic sunflower oil. They also sell a mother's massage oil which is 95 per cent organic ingredients.

Physique Management Company Limited
Jackson Grove
Grove Road
Drayton
Portsmouth
Hampshire
PO6 1UP
Tel: 0870 60 70 381
www.physique.uk.com

Sells a range of shaped massage supports, Fitball and Soft Over Ball for use in pregnancy, Mats and Lisa Westlake Great Expectations pregnancy programme video.

The Baby Catalogue
Sells Noo-Noo's Newborn Massage Oil, which is a nourishing combination of cold pressed carrier oils (olive, grapeseed, coconut and sesame).

They also sell as Sleepytime Sam Massage Oil (for babies 3 months and above) which contains Camomile and Lavender.

Their Joob-Joobs body lotion is a nice alternative to massage oil.

Perfectly Happy People Ltd
31/33 Park Royal Road
London
NW10 7LQ
Tel: 0870 607 0545
www.the babycatalogue.com

Baby Publications
The Local Baby Directory Ltd
(An A–Z of everything for pregnant women, babies and children)
11 Graydon Avenue
Chichester
West Sussex
PO19 2RF
Tel: 020 8742 8724
www.babydirectory.com

Music Classes for Babies & Children (6 weeks up to 3 years)
Mumbaba Ltd
Tel: 01243 3899844

Relaxation Music for Baby Massage

Mother and Baby CD (Mind Body Soul Series)
New World Music Limited
The Barn
Becks Green
St Andrews
Beccles
Suffolk
NR34 8NB
Tel: 01986 781682
E-mail: info@newworldmusic.co.uk.
Website: www.newworldmusic.com

Baby Massage Instructors

To find a qualified instructor of baby massage contact:

The Federation of Holistic Therapists
3rd Floor
Eastleigh House
Eastleigh
Hampshire
SO50 9FD
Tel: 02380 684500
Fax: 02380 651493
www.fht.org.uk

The International Association of Infant Massage Instructors (IAIM)
UK Office
56 Sparsholt Road
Barking
Essex
IG11 7YYQ
Tel:/fax: 020 8591 1399
www.iaim.org.uk
E-mail: mail@iaim.org.uk

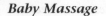

Other Useful Contacts

Sure Start
Level 2
Caxton House
Tothill Street
London
SW1H 9NA
Tel: 020 7273 4830
Fax: 020 7273 5182
www.surestart.gov.uk
E-mail: sure.start~dfee.gov.uk

Aims to promote the physical, intellectual and social development of pre-schoolchildren, particularly those who are disadvantaged, to ensure they are ready to flourish when they enter school.

The National Childbirth Trust
Alexandra House
Oldham Terrace
London
W3 6NH
Tel: 020 89912 8637

Information and support for mothers, including breast-feeding information, antenatal classes, post-natal groups. Write with SAE for details of nearest branch and information pack.

Active Birth Centre
23 Bickerton Road
London
N19 5JT
Tel: 020 7482 5554

Promotes a holistic approach to childbirth. Antenatal and post-natal classes. Publishes a list of UK active birth teachers. Send SAE for details.

Association for Post-natal Illness
25 Jerdan Place
London
SW6 1BE
Tel: 020 7386 0868

Telephone support for mothers suffering from post-natal depression. Send SAE for information pack.

Meet-a-Mum Association
26 Avenue Road
South Norwood
London
SE25 4DX
Tel: 020 8771 5595

Support for mothers suffering from post-natal depression or who feel lonely and isolated looking after a child at home. Will try to put mothers in touch with other mothers with similar problems, or a group of mothers locally. Write with SAE for details of local groups.

Complementary Therapies for Babies

Baby Yoga

The Baby Yoga Company Ltd
PO Box 2616
Great Dunmow
Essex
CM6 1XA
Tel: 01371 873138
Fax: 01371 873382
www.thebabyyogacompany.com
E-mail:info@the babyyogacompany.com

Baby Tui Na

Bodyharmonics Centre
54 Flecker's Drive
Hatherley
Cheltenham
GL51 5BD
Tel: 01242 582168
www.bodyharmonic.co.uk
E-mail: mariamercati@bodyharmonics.co.uk

Cranial Osteopathy

General Council and Register of Osteopaths
56 London Street
Reading
Berks
RG1 4SQ
Tel: 0118 757 6585

British School of Osteopathy
1–4 Suffolk Street
London
SW1Y 4HG
Tel: 020 7930 6093/9254
Fax: 020 7839 1098

Osteopathic Centre for Children
19a Cavendish Square
London
WIM 9AD
Tel: 020 7495 1231

Cranial Osteopathic Association
478 Baker St
Enfield
Middlesex
EN1 3QS
Tel: 020 8367 5561

Flower Essences

The Dr Edward Bach Centre
Mount Vernon
Bakers Lane
Sotwell
Wallingford
Oxfordshire
OX10 OPZ
Tel: 01491 834678
Fax: 01491 825022
www.bachcentre.com

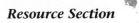

Homeopathy

The British Homeopathic Association
27a Devonshire Street
London
WIG 6PN
Tel: 020 7935 2163

(Medically qualified homeopaths only)

The Society of Homeopaths
4a Artizan Rd
Northampton
NN1 4HU
www.homeopathy.org.uk
E-mail: info@homepathy-soh.org

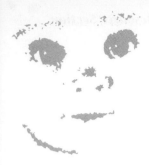

Bibliography and Further Reading

Dr Alan Heath & Nicki Bainbridge
Baby Massage: the Calming Power of Touch
Dorling Kindersley
ISBN 0–7513–0843–9

Peter Walker
The Practical Art of Baby Massage
Carroll & Brown Publishers Limited
ISBN 1–903258–10–3

Vimala McClure
Infant Massage: a handbook for loving parents
Souvenir Press Limited
ISBN 0–285–63617–0

Frederick Leboyer
The Traditional Art of Baby Massage
Newmarket Press
ISBN 1–55704–314–0

Amelia D. Auckett
Baby Massage: Parent–Child Bonding Through Touch
Newmarket Press
ISBN 1–55704–022–2

Kathy Fleming Drehobl, Mary Gengler Fuhr
Paediatric Massage for the Child with Special Needs
Harcourt Health Sciences Company
ISBN 076164092–4

Janet McGregor
Introduction to the Anatomy and Physiology of Children
Routledge
ISBN 0–415–21509–9

Dr Tanvir Jamil & Karen Evennett
The Alternative Pregnancy Handbook
Piatkus
ISBN 0 7499 2117 X

Elaine Stillerman
Mother Massage
Dell Publishing
ISBN 0440–50702–2

Sally K Child
An A–Z of Children's Health
Argyll Publishing
ISBN 1 902831 40

Dr Sally Ward
Baby Talk
Random House Group Limited
ISBN 0 7126 8098 5

Karen Sullivan
Natural Healthcare for Children
Piatkus
ISBN 0–7499–2115–3

Dr Bernard Valman
The British Medical Association Children's Medical Guide
Dorking Kindersley
ISBN 0–780751–0564–2

Richard Landsown and Marjorie Walker
Your Child's Development from birth to adolescence
Frances Lincoln Limited
ISBN 0–7112–1114–0

Marian Bwaver, Jo Brewster, Pauline Jones, Anne Keene, Sally Neaum, Jill Tallack
Babies and Young Children Book 1: Early Years Development (2nd Edition)
ISBN 0–7487–3974–2

Marcia Mercati
Tui Na Massage for a healthier brighter child
Gaia Books Limited
1SBN 1–85675–125–2

T. Berry Brazelton, MD
Touchpoints: your child's emotional and behavioural development
Perseus Publishing
ISBN 0–201–62690–X

Index

Page numbers in italics refer to illustrations. Terms in the index generally refer to the overall topic: baby massage e.g. benefits, outcomes, unless otherwise specified e.g. contra-indications, pregnancy.

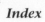